Contributions to Psychology and Medicine

Contributions to Psychology and Medicine

Michel Pierre Janisse
Editor

Individual Differences, Stress, and Health Psychology

With 12 Illustrations

Springer-Verlag
New York Berlin Heidelberg
London Paris Tokyo

Michel Pierre Janisse
Department of Psychology
University of Manitoba
Winnipeg, Manitoba R3T 2N2
Canada

Advisor
J. Richard Eiser
Department of Psychology
Washington Singer Laboratories
University of Exeter
Exeter EX4 4QG
England

Library of Congress Cataloging in Publication Data
Janisse, Michel Pierre.
  Individual differences, stress, and health psychology.
  (Contributions to psychology and medicine)
  Includes bibliographies.
  1. Medicine and psychology. 2. Stress (Psychology)
3. Difference (Psychology) 4. Individuality.
I. Title. II. Series. [DNLM: 1. Behavior. 2. Individuality.
3. Psychophysiologic Disorders. 4. Stress,
Psychological. 5. Type A Personality. WM 90J33i]
R726.5.H4337 1988   616.9′8   87-32192

Typeset by Asco Trade Typesetting Ltd, Hong Kong.
Printed and bound by R.R. Donnelley & Sons, Harrisonburg, Virginia.
Printed in the United States of America.

9 8 7 6 5 4 3 2 1

ISBN 0-387-96669-2 Springer-Verlag New York Berlin Heidelberg
ISBN 3-540-96669-2 Springer-Verlag Berlin Heidelberg New York

To the memory of my mother and sister:

Madelyn Philomene Janisse
and
Janis Lecadie Janisse

Preface

This book emerges from two sources. The first was my attempt to understand how individual differences lead to the multiplicity of reactions people display to stressors and in stressful situations, particularly as related to health and illness. The second was the opportunity to bring together in one volume at least some of the experts in the field to discuss their research focusing on these issues. Hence, a book designed to shed some light on the relationships among individual differences, stress, and health psychology.

Health Psychology (and the related field of Behavioral Medicine) are currently among the most productive areas in the behavioral and life sciences. Eminent scientists in such fields as cardiology, epidemiology, medicine, psychiatry, psychology, physiology, and other biological, behavioral, and social science disciplines are devoting more and more of their scholarly efforts to the development of an understanding of the interaction among individual differences, stress, and health. The emergence of Health Psychology as an identifiable discipline in the last 15 years has been accompanied by the birth of about half a dozen new journals on the topic, several books devoted to exploring aspects of it, and countless journal articles appearing in both North American and international periodicals.

The present volume is an attempt to offer readers what some of the best minds in the area have to say about the *integration* of individual differences and stress within this new field of Health Psychology. The goal of bringing together distinguished international researchers in the field resulted in this presentation of their latest research findings. In addition, they speculate on the future of the field, particularly on its application to developing treatments or changes in lifestyles that may prevent or alleviate such disorders as cancer, coronary heart disease, hypertension, and posttraumatic stress syndrome.

The book is organized into eight chapters that focus on aspects of the relationship suggested by the wording in the title, *Individual Differences, Stress, and Health Psychology*. The first chapter is an overview by Rosenman of the known effects of anxiety and other emotions on cardiovascular disorders. He provides an orientation to some of the basic issues in the field of Health Psychology and a review of the literature as background to the rest of the book. The second chapter, by Endler, serves a similar function for anxiety, as he reviews the history of the concept and provides a wide-ranging review/ commentary on his own interactional approach to anxiety. In the next four chapters, authors deal with specific individual difference constructs and discuss how these are related to both health and illness. In Chapter 3, Janisse and Dyck review some of the psychological and physiological aspects of the Type A behavior pattern and their implications for theory, focusing particularly on the notions of exaggerated physiological responsivity, the importance of controlling the environment, and hostility reactions as important factors to be considered in future theory and research on this behavior pattern. Chapter 4, by Zuckerman, concentrates on the literature pertaining to the concept of risk taking/sensation seeking as it relates to health concerns, with a particular focus on smoking behavior. Spielberger, Krasner, and Solomon, in Chapter 5, review the role of the anger-hostility-aggression complex in health-related areas, and argue persuasively for the need to measure both the direction of anger expression (in or out) and the extent of an individual's ability to control anger. In Chapter 6, Sarason provides a brief history of the concept of social support and its historical relationship to both health and recovery, followed by an exposition of his recent research on the effects of both life events and social support as related to coping with stress. In Chapter 7, Eysenck presents the reader with a broad review of personality correlates of both cancer and cardiovascular disorders, followed by an explication of two large-scale studies (in Germany and Yugoslavia) that strikingly demonstrate the psychological differences between victims of these two disorders. The final chapter, by Strelau, presents his intriguing theory of temperament as a base for the understanding and explanation of individual differences in reactions to stress and consequent behaviors when unable to cope.

It is to be expected, as with any book of edited papers, that individual readers of this volume may adjudge the contributions to be of varying interest and of varying relevance to their own endeavors. To aid the reader, an attempt has been made to link each of the chapters with brief interstitial material that both previews the coming chapter and provides some perspective to its relation to the rest of the book.

The idea and fashioning of this book were not the work of just one person. In addition to the contributors, several persons have provided invaluable assistance in putting this work together. Cynthia Erickson has been my number one assistant from the beginning of this project, some 3 years ago. Along the way we have been ably assisted by Cindy Cain and all of the secretarial pool in the Department of Psychology at the University of Manitoba.

I would also like to extend my gratitude to current and former graduate students who are inspirations as well as assistants: Atholl T. Malcolm, Nukte Edguer, and Dieter Schonwetter. Finally my friend and colleague, Dennis G. Dyck, has continued to supply me with ample portions of his prodigious energy and intelligence. Also, for adding their support to this project, I am deeply grateful to John Finlay, Dean of Arts, University of Manitoba; Sheila Brown, Dean of Human Ecology, University of Manitoba; G. Ron Norton, Head, Department of Psychology, University of Winnipeg; the Psychological Association of Manitoba; and the Manitoba Psychological Society.

MICHEL PIERRE JANISSE

Contents

Contributors

DENNIS G. DYCK, Ph.D.
Department of Psychology, University of Manitoba, Winnipeg,
Manitoba, Canada R3T 2N2

NORMAN S. ENDLER, Ph.D.
Department of Psychology, York University, North York, Ontario,
Canada M3J 1P3

HANS J. EYSENCK, D.Sc.
Institute of Psychiatry, University of London, London SE5 8AF,
United Kingdom

MICHEL PIERRE JANISSE, Ph.D.
Department of Psychology, University of Manitoba, Winnipeg,
Manitoba, Canada R3T 2N2

SUSAN S. KRASNER, M.A.
Center for Research in Behavioral Medicine and Health Psychology,
University of South Florida, Tampa, Florida, 33620-8100 USA

RAY H. ROSENMAN, M.D.
SRI International, 333 Ravenswood Avenue, Menlo Park, California,
94025 USA

IRWIN G. SARASON, Ph.D.
Department of Psychology, NI-25, University of Washington, Seattle,
Washington, 98195 USA

ELDRA P. SOLOMON, M.A.
Center for Research in Behavioral Medicine and Health Psychology,
University of South Florida, Tampa, Florida, 33620-8100 USA

CHARLES D. SPIELBERGER, Ph.D.
Center for Research in Behavioral Medicine and Health Psychology,
University of South Florida, Tampa, Florida, 33620-8100 USA

JAN STRELAU, Ph.D.
Faculty of Psychology, University of Warsaw, 00-183 Warsaw, Poland

MARVIN ZUCKERMAN, Ph.D.
Department of Psychology, University of Delaware, Newark, Delaware,
19716 USA

1

The Impact of Certain Emotions in Cardiovascular Disorders

Ray H. Rosenman

In this first chapter, Rosenman begins with a brief review of the voluminous literature relating cardiovascular disease and various emotions—and the history is quite long indeed. The chapter also provides a historical orientation to the material in the rest of the book. Rosenman reviews the known links between cardiac arrhythmias and sudden cardiac death, noting that the presence of stress often precedes the onset of these disorders. He argues that the effects of stress upon blood pressure, and hence hypertension in humans, are really not very well understood and at best the direct effects of stress and anxiety are most likely transitory rather than long lasting. Such environmental factors are said to have their effects in interactions with other variables such as genetic predispositions. Specific attention is also paid to the relationship of anger to hypertension, focusing on the role of unexpressed hostility as an associated factor. Lifestyle habits also come under scrutiny here, as the effects upon cardiovascular health of alcohol, nicotine, and caffeine are reviewed. The effects of anxiety upon sleep and its consequent impact upon the cardiovascular system are also considered. It is argued that the common overuse of the defense mechanism of denial by Type A individuals in suppressing symptoms may result in a delay in seeking medical care and hence have adverse health consequences. On the other hand, the use of denial to subdue anxiety and its beta-adrenergic stimulation has led to improved survival rates in some cardiac patients. The chapter also contains a thorough review of individual difference factors in mitral valve prolapse as well as the role of the Type A behavior pattern risk factor in ischemic heart disease.

—EDITOR

Interrelationships between emotions and the cardiovascular system have held a long and unique place in clinical medicine, particularly the relationship of anxiety to cardiovascular symptoms, culminating in the recent emphasis on the association of anxiety syndromes to mitral valve prolapse (MVP). Physicians have long accepted a relationship between emotions and transient cardiovascular responses and symptoms. In 1628 Harvey (Burchell, 1984; Harvey, 1984) stated that "Every affection of the mind that is attended with either pain or pleasure, hope or fear, is the cause of an agitation whose influence extends to the heart." John C. Williams distinguished nervous palpitations from organic disease in his 1836 text (Williams, 1836). The functional nature of cardiovascular symptoms associated with anxiety was emphasized by DaCosta in 1871 (DaCosta, 1871), based on his observations of the irritable heart syndrome occurring in Civil War soldiers. MacLean made similar observations in British soldiers in 1867 (MacLean, 1867). George Beard supported the concept of functional cardiovascular disorders by introducing the term neurasthenia in 1867 (Beard, 1867); its international use followed, to be replaced by neurocirculatory asthenia and the subsequent anxiety neurosis of World War I, systolic click syndrome in the 1960s, and current emphasis on hyperdynamic beta-adrenergic dysfunction in anxiety disorders and symptomatic MVP.

Around 200 BC Hippocrates said, "Let no one persuade you to cure the headache until he has first given you his soul to be cured. For this is the great error of our day in the treatment of the human body, that physicians separate the soul from the body." The brain/heart dichotomy has resulted in part from difficulties in definition and quantitation of emotions. For example, subjective anxiety is difficult to define. In the United States, one descriptive word is used, whereas in most European languages there are two words (Lader, 1984), main roots being derived from the Latin "angor," referring to transitory physical symptoms, and "anxietas," denoting a predisposition to mental disquiet, uncertainty, and fear. A greater interest between emotions and cardiovascular disorders has been promulgated by relationships to hypertension and ischemic heart disease. The association of anxiety disorders with MVP has stimulated a more unified interest among cardiologists and psychiatrists because symptomatic MVP patients may initially seek advice either for physical symptoms or for emotional manifestations of the anxiety states that are often associated with MVP.

A different relationship between emotions and the cardiovascular system was emphasized by Osler (1892) in the late 19th century when he observed that his typical patient with ischemic heart disease was ". . . a man whose engine is always set at full speed ahead." In the 1950s, evidence began to accumulate that the Type A behavior pattern (TABP) may play an important role in the pathogenesis of ischemic heart disease (Rosenman, 1983; Rosenman & Chesney, 1982).

The present discussion only highlights some relationships between emotions and cardiovascular disorders. In this association, physicians may first recall a role of emotions in cardiac arrhythmias.

Arrhythmias

Autonomic cardiac nerves are driven by preganglionic sympathic neurons in the spinal cord, and these are under control of descending brain pathways. A major source of background autonomic nervous system activity thus depends on the integrity of neurons that drive sympathetic nervous system centers that are part of contiguous adrenergic neurons. Central stimuli that increase sympathetic neural traffic and that suppress baroreflex activity usually produce a rise of blood pressure and heart rate and increased release of epinephrine, while vagal nerve activity is inhibited. During the post-stimulus period the blood pressure usually remains briefly elevated, baroreflexes are no longer inhibited, and vagal excitation occurs. It is this vulnerable period of increased vagal tone and residual sympathetic neural drive that may underlie the occurrence of ventricular arrhythmias after exercise (Lown, 1979).

Sudden Cardiac Death

The post-stimulus period is relevant to the problem of sudden cardiac death, which almost invariably is due to ventricular fibrillation (Skinner, Lie, & Entman, 1975). The pathophysiology of sudden death is not merely coronary artery disease (Lown, 1979), but best comprehended as an electrophysiologic abnormality manifested as electrical instability of the myocardium (MEI). MEI provides the substrate upon which a triggering factor can precipitate ventricular fibrillation, and this often is adrenergic stimulation (Lown & Verrier, 1976). Both MEI and triggering catecholamine input are related to higher nervous system activity (Lown, 1979). Much of our knowledge in this regard stems from studies done in experimental animals (Lown & Verrier, 1976; Skinner, 1985). In unanesthetized animals, ligation of a coronary artery does not result in ventricular fibrillation if psychological stress is eliminated (Skinner, Lie, & Entman, 1975)—or, in the presence of such stress, if a cerebral pathway is blocked that connects the frontal cortex to the autonomic nuclei in the brainstem (Skinner & Reed, 1981). MEI is increased in animals by an anxiety-fear-anger response such as occurs in a totally restrained dog when another dog is brought into the laboratory setting. Repetitive ventricular ectopy does not trigger ventricular fibrillation in such restrained dogs unless the MEI is first increased by the psychological stressor.

In humans, an increased MEI is induced by overt or silent myocardial ischemia and higher neural traffic can precipitate ventricular fibrillation in patients with coronary artery disease. Important triggering factors often relate to neurophysiologic activity that occurs in response to psychological stresses (Lown & Verrier, 1976; Skinner, 1985). Coronary artery vasospasm and platelet aggregation may also play a role.

The vulnerable period of the cardiac cycle occurs in the brief interval at the apex of the upright T wave in the electrocardiogram, when a normal patchwork of inhomogeneous electrical activity is present because of a variable recovery time of fibers during repolarization. Acute myocardial infarction or other autonomic stimulation can reduce the threshold during the vulnerable period, with an enhanced susceptibility to fibrillation in the conducting myocardial fibers (Lown & Verrier, 1976; Lown, 1979).

There are many anecdotal reports that link sudden cardiac death with profound emotions (Skinner, 1985). Reich and associates (Reich, deSilva, Lown, & Murawski, 1981) found that a high number of emotionally stressful events had occurred in successfully resuscitated patients in proximate relationships to the occurrence of their ventricular arrhythmias, including interpersonal conflicts, bereavement, threatened or actual marital separation, public humiliation, loss in vocational life, or other sources of major anxiety. This relationship was observed to occur more frequently in persons exhibiting Type A behavior by Bruhn and colleagues (1984) and there is evidence that Type A subjects with ischemic heart disease are more prone to exhibit ventricular ectopy (Jennings & Follansbee, 1984).

The role of higher neural traffic in the genesis of lethal arrhythmias is now firmly based on much evidence that links emotionally stressful events and sudden cardiac death in both animals and humans (Lown & Verrier, 1976; Bruhn et al., 1984). Autonomic neural activity can induce ventricular ectopy and lower the threshold to ventricular fibrillation (Skinner & Reed, 1981). Sudden death occurs more frequently in males than in females, plausibly related to the greater male catecholamine response to stressors (Frankenhaeuser, 1982). In patients with myocardial ischemia, relatively minor physical or emotional stress can precipitate sudden cardiac death (Reich et al., 1981; Schwartz, 1984). However, in a small proportion of subjects it would appear that extreme adrenergic stimulation can trigger sudden death in the absence of coronary artery disease and this can be induced by severe emotional stress (Reich et al., 1981; Schwartz, 1984) or prolonged physical exertion (Vuori, Makarainen, & Jaaskelainen, 1978).

In females who suffer sudden cardiac death, there is often a history of psychiatric disorders, of taking psychotropic drugs, or of being cigarette smokers (Talbott, Kuller, & Perper, 1981), all of which are associated with enhanced autonomic activity. A synergistic effect can be induced by caffeine or nicotine, which are known to reduce the fibrillatory threshold (Hennekens, Lown, Rosener, Grufferman, & Dalen, 1980). Such sensitizing substances are capable of increasing the deleterious influences of stress-induced stimulation of autonomic neural traffic (Dembroski, MacDougall, Cardozo, & Krug-Fite, 1985).

In view of the increased MEI associated with environmental stress responses (Lown & Verrier, 1976), it is not surprising that long-term mortality in post-infarction patients is found to be strongly related to such psychosocial factors as higher degree of adverse life circumstances and social isolation (Ruberman, Weinblatt, & Goldberg, 1984).

The predisposition to sudden cardiac death is enhanced in subjects with depletion of body potassium (Nordrehaug, 1985). Activation of beta-2 adrenoreceptors increases potassium entry into cells, thereby acutely decreasing serum potassium (Brown, 1985; Brown, Brown, & Murphy, 1983). When this already has been decreased by the use of diuretic therapy in hypertensive subjects, the risk of ventricular fibrillation during acute myocardial ischemia is further increased (Dyckner, Helmers, & Wester, 1984).

The presence of left ventricular hypertrophy (LVH) also increases the risk of sudden cardiac death in hypertensive patients (Schatzkin, Cupples, Neeren, Morelock, & Kannel, 1984). Although LVH is related in part to an increased afterload on the heart, a thickened left ventricular wall can be found in young offspring of hypertensive parents prior to any sustained elevation of the blood pressure (Culpepper, Sodt, Messerli, Ruschhaupt, & Arcilla, 1983). In progeny who are thus genetically predisposed to hypertension, this early myocardial thickening appears to be causally related to an enhanced noradrenergic secretion that contributes to the development of LVH (Trimarco et al., 1985).

Hypertension

The relationship of anxiety to hypertension remains unclear. The central nervous system is critically involved in regulation of the blood pressure and integrates information from both the organism and the environment in order to provide neurohormonal adjustments that are essential to maintenance of the blood pressure. One major hypothesis (Chesney, 1986) suggests that environmental factors such as psychosocial stressors may stimulate autonomic overactivity that increases cardiovascular responses and elevates the blood pressure (Krakoff, Dziedzic, Mann, Felton, & Yaeger, 1985). This hypothesis is based upon well accepted facts concerned with neurohormonal circulatory regulation. Thus, blood pressure can be increased by activation of higher neural sites with neuroanatomic connections to the sympathetic nervous system and many of these sites connect with higher centers that are involved in the perception of the environment. Considerable data indicate that external stressors are capable of elevating arterial blood pressure via neurohormonal mechanisms (Diamond, 1982). Studies in animals support the hypothesis that certain types of stress can induce elevated blood pressure (Henry & Stephens, 1977). However, when the stressor is removed, sustained hypertension is the exception. In 1956 a Task Force concluded (Brody et al., 1987) that there was inadequate evidence to support the belief that stress alone can induce sustained hypertension in otherwise healthy animals, but that hypertension can occur more readily in response to environmental stressors in animals that are predisposed by reason of genetic forces, salt ingestion, or decreased renal mass.

The data concerning a stress-blood pressure relationship in humans are even less clear. Stress can elevate blood pressure in humans, but, as in animals, sustained hypertension infrequently is observed when the stressor is removed. For example, the rise of blood pressure observed in combat soldiers generally returns to normal when they are removed from active combat. Changing cultural norms from a more primitive to more complex level may be associated with a rise of blood pressure (Salmond, Joseph, Prior, Stanley, & Wessen, 1985), but this probably involves an interaction of dietary and psychosocial factors. An enhanced pressor response to external stressors can occur in offspring of hypertensive parents (Falkner, Onesti, Angelakos, Fernandez, & Langman, 1974). Predisposing factors such as genetic forces, salt ingestion, and renal disease appear necessary for the reliable expression of stress-induced hypertension in both animals and humans (Brody et al., 1987).

Much of the evidence that underlies the belief in a causal relationship of stress factors to hypertension is based on studies of acute responses, such as in the enhanced cardiovascular response to stressors that occurs in some offspring of hypertensive parents (Falkner et al., 1974). Nevertheless, there is a widespread belief that anxiety is causally related to sustained hypertension, which itself can affect behavior at anatomic, physiologic, and emotional levels. Many antihypertensive drugs and even the diagnosis of hypertension can induce anxiety and other behavioral responses (Elias & Streeten, 1980). Moreover, hypertensive individuals have alterations of physiological function that interact with behavioral factors (Elias & Streeten, 1980), further clouding a relationship between anxiety and hypertension.

Plasma catecholamine levels tend to be higher in many hypertensive patients (Cottier, Shapiro, & Julius, 1984), and heightened autonomic neural traffic may alter emotions and behaviors. This may particularly be observed in younger persons with labile blood pressures or mild hypertension (Esler et al., 1977). An indication of the deleterious effects of sympathetic overactivity may be seen in the improved test performance scores that can follow administration of beta-adrenergic blocking agents. The ability of such agents to dampen manifestations of anxiety is well known to public speakers, musicians, and even some athletes (Taggart, Carruthers, & Somerville, 1973).

An enhanced pressor response to psychological stressors that occurs in some hypertensive subjects and their offspring may have a genetic basis. Young hyperreactors more often progress to sustained hypertension (Falkner, Onesti, & Hamstra, 1981). But this is an inconsistent finding and hypertensive subjects also are not consistently more reactive to stressors compared to normotensive individuals. Subjects with Type A behavior generally respond to external stressors with enhanced cardiovascular reactivity compared to Type B subjects (Rosenman & Chesney, 1982), but Type A and B persons do not exhibit any difference in their prevalence of sustained hypertension (Rosenman & Chesney, 1982; Shekelle, Schoenberger, & Stamler, 1976). The variability of the blood pressure observed in the daily milieu by ambulatory monitoring procedures does not correlate with the severity or duration of hypertension and there is little support for the concept of increased variability among persons with borderline elevations of the blood pressure (Conway, 1983). The variability during ambulatory monitoring is similar in subjects who have normal blood pressures with mild or marked elevation (Pickering, Harshfield, Kleinert, Blank, & Laragh, 1982). Nor are there any population-based studies that show that hyperreactive normotensives exhibit an increased likelihood for sustained hypertension. There is, therefore, inadequate evidence to indicate that stress-induced rise of the blood pressure is a causal precursor of sustained hypertension (Conway, 1983). Stress-induced cardiovascular reactivity can be considered to be a correlate or marker for the risk of developing hypertension, while not necessarily being its cause (Rosenman, 1985).

Anger and Hypertension

The effect of anxiety on the blood pressure is probably of more transient nature, rather than having a significant causal role in the pathogenesis of sustained hypertension. Relaxation-type therapy may provide some benefits for a small number of hypertensive subjects but may not be well directed at the pathogenesis of the elevated blood pressure in most hypertensive patients. More important in this regard may be an association of the blood pressure level with dimensions of hostility and anger (Chesney, 1986; Diamond, 1982; Rosenman, 1985; Schwartz, Weinberger, & Singer, 1981). A large number of studies have found that many hypertensive patients exhibit unexpressed hostility, and that resting blood pressure levels as well as sustained elevations are associated with self-reported ineffective management of anger (Diamond, 1982). During ambulatory monitoring in the daily milieu, the variability of the blood pressure is found to be correlated with the level of hostility (Pickering et al., 1982). In the laboratory setting, exaggerated and more prolonged pressor responses to a variety of stressful cognitive stimuli occur in hypertensive persons who exhibit unexpressed hostility and anger (Baer, Collins, Bourenoff, & Ketchel, 1979). Moreover, offspring of hypertensive parents who progress to sustained hypertension are more often those who show exaggerated pressor responses to stressors that are designed to elicit anger. Among such subjects, an enhanced risk for sustained hypertension is found in those who have the greatest difficulty in expressing such induced anger (Falkner, Onesti, & Hamstra, 1981). It would thus appear that the blood pressure level and risk for sustained elevation are far better correlated with ineffective anger management and expression than with the level of anxiety. This has led to the recent change of emphasis in some behavioral approaches to the treatment of hypertensive patients (Chesney, 1986; Rosenman, 1985).

Habits

Consideration of the role of anxiety in cardiovascular disorders should extend to the fact that it is related to various habits that affect the cardiovascular systems. It can only be mentioned that diet and weight are related to serum lipids, blood pressure, and ischemic heart disease. Alcohol has a more complex relationship. Considerable evidence has accumulated to confirm a relationship of moderate alcohol consumption to reduced incidence of ischemic heart disease in population-based as well as prospective studies (Marmot, 1984), despite the adverse effects of alcohol ingestion on the blood pressure level of hypertensive subjects (Klatsky, Friedman, Siegelaum, & Gerad, 1977). There is good evidence for an interaction between drinking habits and life events. Moreover, studies of in-patients who are being treated for alcohol detoxification indicate a high prevalence of anxiety disorders (Weiss & Rosenberg, 1985). Stressful events are less strongly related to symptoms among moderate alcohol drinkers than among either abstainers or those who heavily ingest alcohol (Neff, 1984), suggesting that its moderate consumption has a stress-buffering role (Neff, 1984; Strahlendorf & Strahlendorf, 1981).

Cigarette smoking also may provide a stress-buffering role for anxiety in some persons but has additive effects with external stress on autonomic neural traffic and associated cardiovascular responses (Dembroski et al., 1985). Both caffeine and nicotine increase locus ceruleus function and therefore may be anxiogenic. Accordingly, although smoking may be used by some to buffer anxiety, it is probably used by others to stimulate arousal (see Zuckerman, Chapter 4).

The acute administration of caffeine causes a modest increase of plasma catecholamines with an associated increase of heart rate and blood pressure, and may affect mood and sleep patterns (Robertson et al., 1978). The pressor response may not solely be due to an effect on catecholamines because it can occur independently, as well as in subjects with autonomic dysfunction (Curatolo & Robertson, 1983). On the other hand, chronic caffeine ingestion probably has little effect on either catecholamines or cardiovascular responses (Curatolo & Robertson, 1983). Stimulation of cardiac arrhythmias by caffeine generally depends on the underlying presence of myocardial ischemia, other cardiovascular disorders such as mitral valve prolapse, or anxiety states in which there may be a hypersensitivity to its adrenergic-stimulating effects. Caffeine has no confirmed effects on either serum lipids or the incidence of ischemic heart disease, and discrepant findings with the scientific literature may largely reflect differences in chronic habits between subjects and controls (Curatolo & Robertson, 1983).

Anxiety has an effect on sleep patterns that is both direct and indirect, through influences on consumption of food, alcohol, caffeine, and nicotine. In subjects with ischemic heart disease, acute coronary events may be prone to occur at times of sleep deprivation, with the associated fatigue and exhaustion that may occur at time of anxiety. Although this important factor is often ignored by physicians, there is ample reason to emphasize this in cardiac patients (Nixon, 1982).

Anxiety and Cardiovascular Disease

The link between anxiety and cardiovascular disease is exemplified in several types of patients. The first is a patient whose problem is mainly anxiety associated with somatic symptoms that suggest heart disease. A second is a patient who is healthy and not anxious but who develops symptoms that are interpreted as being due to heart disease. A third is a patient with minor heart disease that is complicated by major anxiety, and a fourth is a patient with major heart disease who develops secondary anxiety. The relationship of anxiety to anginal symptoms is well known. Among patients awaiting bypass graft surgery, the frequency and severity of anginal symptoms are related far more to psychological and behavioral factors such as disturbed sleep, distressed responses, life dissatisfaction, and hostile dimensions than they are to the severity of the coronary artery disease (Jenkins, Stanton, Klein, Savageau, & Harken, 1983).

The link between anxiety and illness is documented in postinfarction patients. Anxiety occurs in most and may be more than mild in at least half of them (Cassem & Hackett, 1977). Most postinfarction patients face difficult adjustments to a loss of status, threat of dependency, changed family and vocational relationships, and fear of death. In Type A patients, anxiety may result from the threat of loss of control over their environments. There is a predictable progression of the psychological responses to myocardial infarction that probably involves anxiety, depression, denial, and convalescence (Cassem & Hackett, 1977; Gentry, Balder, Oude-Weme, Musch, & Gary, 1983). Type A individuals appear to employ a greater denial and suppression of symptoms that enable them to endure stress at higher levels and for longer intervals, compared to those with Type B behavior. This type of denial may lead to delay in seeking medical care after onset of symptoms, with adverse consequences for immediate survival. However, denial is a coping mechanism that is used to suppress anxiety and its associated beta-adrenergic stimulation (Gentry et al., 1983) and this in turn may lead to an improved subsequent rate of survival. Type A patients in the coronary care unit are observed to be more alert, active, friendly, competitive, emotionally withdrawn, and concerned about their return to work and family control than are Type B patients. They display greater initiative in their daily hospital care, are prone to take charge of the situation which they soon regard as a challenge to be overcome, and they tend to be discharged earlier from the hospital (Gentry et al., 1983).

The Western Collaborative Group Study (WCGS) is a prospective study of 3,154 middle-aged males employed in 10 companies in California (Rosenman et al., 1964). They were followed from 1960 to 1969, during which time 257 of the initially healthy men suffered the occurrence of ischemic heart disease. After multivariate adjustment for other risk factors, subjects who were assessed at intake as exhibiting Type A behavior were found to have a twofold higher incidence of coronary heart disease, compared to participants adjudged to exhibit the converse Type B behavior pattern (Rosenman, Brand, Sholtz, & Friedman, 1976). A mortality follow-up 22 years after intake into the study found that among men who survived their initial coronary event, those who were Type A appeared to have a more favorable long-term rate of survival than did Type B subjects. This finding supports the belief that denial may lead to a reduced impact on physiological and behavioral health outcomes (Cassem & Hackett, 1977; Gentry et al., 1983), perhaps to the extent that an illness is perceived to have predictable factors that are controllable. It is possible that the cognitive process of denial reduces anxiety manifestations otherwise associated with enhanced autonomic neural traffic that has adverse consequences for the recurrence of both fatal and nonfatal events.

Mitral Valve Prolapse

Although the role of anxiety in cardiovascular disorders has long been of interest in clinical medicine, it assumes a new importance with its relevance for the pathogenesis of mitral valve prolapse (MVP). Symptomatic MVP may be a paradigm of the interaction of physical and psychological variables. Anxiety has long been viewed in psychological terms that convey an image of overreaction to life stress, hypochondriasis, and hysteria, with labels such as hyperventilation syndrome, hypoglycemia, neurasthenia, functional cardiovascular disorders, irritable heart syndrome, soldier's heart, effort syndrome, and neurocirculatory asthenia. It is probable that many patients thus diagnosed in the past would now be adjudged to have suffered from a biological anxiety disorder that is associated with high prevalence of MVP. Although well identified as a clinical entity only two decades ago, MVP has emerged as the most common valvular disorder in the United States (Dean, 1985). The recognition of its frequent association with anxiety disorders has led to a more unified interest in the brain/heart relationship. Patients with MVP are sometimes confusing because manifestations of their associated anxiety disorder are perceived as neurotic, a label that may have led to long-term, adverse consequences.

MVP refers to the invagination or herniation of the mitral valve leaflets into the left atrium during ventricular systole. Although considered by some to be a specific syndrome, the variability of findings indicates that it has multiple causes. The mitral valve is a complex structure and its proper function depends on the integrity of components that include the left atrium, fibrous annulus, valve leaflets, chordae tendineae, papillary muscles, and supporting structures at the base of the papillary muscles. Abnormality of any part can lead to a failure of leaflet coaptation. Under the burden of left ventricular (LV) contraction, prolapsed valve cusps can stretch and become concave toward the left atrium and take on a pleated or scalloped appearance, while an increased tugging effect on the chordae leads to their elongation and thinning, and the annulus dilates. This can be associated with mitral regurgitation, and in some can eventuate in a ballooning, billowing, or floppy valve.

MVP can occur with histologically normal valve leaflets, occurring secondarily as the result of dysfunction of one or more components of the mitral apparatus. Thus, it can be associated with ischemia or infarction of the papillary muscles, disordered LV contractility that occurs with myocardial infarction, aneurysm, or cardiomyopathies, and with myocardial ischemia that results from obstructive or vasoconstrictive coronary artery disease.

Idiopathic MVP occurs as the result of histological abnormalities of the leaflets, the basic defect being xyomatous degeneration. The dense fibrous core is replaced by loose myxomatous tissue rich in acid mucopolysaccharides and the chordae are often similarly involved. It has been postulated that the myxomatous transformation is due to a genetic defect of DNA that results in mesodermal production of faulty mesenchymal tissue from which connective tissue is derived. As the valve support loses its integrity, the leaflets become stretched and elongated, the chordae attenuate and elongate, the annulus dilates, and the leaflets become overly large relative to left ventricle size, allowing the valve to prolapse as the systolic ejection shrinks the ventricular volume below a critical level. In support of this hypothesis is the fact that MVP occurs with increased frequency in patients with inherited disorders of connective tissue as well as in subjects with thoracic skeletal and other noncardiac characteristics that could have originated in the mesoderm. MVP is thus more prone to occur in individuals with a smaller thoracic cage due to a narrow antero-posterior diameter, straight back, pectus excavatum, scoliosis, or kyphoscoliosis (Salomon, Shah, & Heinle, 1975). It has been pointed out that the primordia of the bony thorax, vertebral column, and fingerprints undergo differentiation in the mesoderm at the same time as the primordia of the mitral valve, during the 35th to 42nd day of fetal development.

Although there is evidence of a collagen abnormality in which its dissolution or dysgenesis in the contiguous pars fibrosa and chordae may lead to ballooning of the leaflets, convincing proof of a genetic mechanism is lacking and no chromosomal abnormality has yet been identified for MVP. It is prone to occur in lean female subjects, and as associated hypomastia, may simply be due to a reduced contribution of adipose tissue to breast size. Although MVP occurs in patients with generalized connective tissue dis-

orders in which structural weakness of the mitral apparatus can lead to prolapse, the majority of subjects with MVP do not exhibit other congenital
defects and the pattern of autosomal dominant inheritance with age- and
sex-dependent expressions (Devereux, Brown, Kramer-Fox, & Laragh,
1982) can be otherwise explained.

The motion of the anterior mitral leaflet is restricted because it abuts the
interventricular septum during diastole and the normal leaflets are displaced
posteriorly into the left atrium. When the LV cavity is disproportionately
small, as in hypertrophic cardiomyopathies, severe pulmonary hypertension,
and secundum-type interatrial septal defects, MVP can occur because the
small LV cavity is unable to accommodate the normal leaflet motion. It has
become apparent that MVP also can occur functionally in the presence of
a disproportionately small LV in the absence of heart disease.

The predilection for prolapse of the posterior leaflet, and in particular of
its middle scallop, supports consideration of a wear and tear phenomenon
rather than a primary collagen abnormality. This and superimposed glyco-
saminoglycan infiltration that gives the valve its myxomatous appearance can
develop in a valve that initially was structurally and histologically normal,
but becomes prolapsed by factors that altered the mechanical forces acting
on the mitral apparatus. Some have considered that the myxomatous transformation in the leaflets and chordae may occur secondarily in response to
catecholamines. The constant stimulation with neuroamines over years may
cause a breakdown of the fibrosa that leads to secondary histologic changes
and normal valves have been shown to produce a factor that appears to
accelerate degradation of the intracellular valve matrix (Feldman et al.,
1985). The fact that patients with MVP commonly exhibit increased
adrenergic stimulation (Boudoulas, Reynolds, Mazzaferri, & Wooley, 1983)
supports a belief that idiopathic MVP that occurs in the absence of other
connective tissue disorders originates as a functional failure of leaflet coaptation, with secondary degenerative histological changes, rather than
being a primary inherited mesenchymal defect. Moreover, the histological
abnormalities observed at autopsy or in surgically excised valves do not
indicate the pathogenesis of MVP.

MVP is commonly observed to occur in young female subjects as a transient phenomenon at a certain stage in life (Savage et al., 1983). There is a
greatly increased prevalence in young adult females that progressively diminishes after their forties. Such observations strongly suggest that MVP is not
primarily due to genetic structural valve abnormalities but to a functional
mechanism that may either be evanescent or more sustained and eventuate
in secondary histologic changes, ballooning, and other complications.

It is now apparent that any disturbance of the normal balance between LV
and mitral valvular size may cause a failure of leaflet coaptation and anatomical prolapse in the absence of initial pathological changes in the valve
apparatus. In particular this may occur when diminished LV cavity size
prevents maintenance of normal leaflet position and contour during ventricu-

lar systole. A disproportion between the mitral valve apparatus and LV cavity size can occur as the result of hemodynamic factors concerned with LV systolic volume and/or contractility, and subjects with MVP often exhibit both subnormal volume and increased contractility associated with beta-adrenergic stimulation. The predisposition for occurrence of MVP in young females is probably in part due to their smaller LV size, compared to males.

The overlap and prolapse of mitral leaflets is associated with a non-ejection systolic click and/or murmur that are respectively usually heard in mid- and late systole. Their relationship to hemodynamic factors explains why such auscultatory phenomena may be intermittent (Savage et al., 1983), as well as the ability of maneuvers that alter ventricular volume and size to change their timing in the cardiac cycle and even cause their temporary disappearance. They are most prominent in the upright position because of the increased beta-adrenergic response to standing.

The belief that a hemodynamic mechanism underlies idiopathic MVP is strongly supported by the fact that it occurs with high prevalence in hyperthyroid patients (Channick et al., 1981). Hyperthyroid patients have an increased density of beta-adrenergic receptors in the myocardium (Feldman et al., 1985) which is associated with an increase of beta-adrenergically mediated LV contractility. The augmented responsiveness of myocardial beta-adrenergic receptors enhances inotropic and chronotropic myocardial activity, with enhanced tugging at chordae that pulls down the posterior leaflet and causes it to overlap and prolapse in the absence of primary histologic changes.

Symptomatic patients with MVP may exhibit increased levels of plasma catecholamines (Boudoulas et al., 1983). However, an increase of plasma norepinephrine may only be a secondary and passive phenomenon. Some symptomatic patients with MVP exhibit a dual dysfunction that involves both the adrenergic and parasympathetic system. Dysautonomic responses are not due to an abnormality of peripheral receptors, but to an abnormal central modulation of baroreflexes that leads to a relative failure of the fine-graded responses that make the autonomic nervous system function in a smooth and stable fashion. Although some believe that MVP may be due to an inherited defect in the central ANS, there is a lack of supporting evidence. Thus the increase of plasma catecholamines is observed to occur only during the daytime milieu, and particularly involves an increased release of epinephrine.

MVP appears to be transmitted in families in an autosomal dominant pattern of inheritance, with age- and sex-dependent expressions (Devereux, Brown, Kramer-Fox et al., 1982). However, there is a parallel pattern of inheritance for height and leanness, and subjects with MVP tend to be taller and to weigh less with a striking relationship to leanness. The inherited factor that predisposes to MVP may merely be a somatotype that is associated with less weight for height, and that also is associated with an augmented beta-adrenergically mediated response to stressors and particularly to orthostatic stress, because the latter is expected to occur in such persons. Subjects with MVP are prone to exhibit lower blood pressures (Devereux, Brown, & Lutas, 1982; Savage et al., 1983). This can probably be ascribed to their somatotypically enhanced beta-adrenergically mediated vasodilation and reduced peripheral resistance. Although an increase of epinephrine occurs in response to all types of stress in patients with MVP, it particularly occurs in the erect position in response to a fall of cardiac output. Rather than being considered to be a hyperkinetic orthostatic response (Frohlich, Kozul, Tarazi, & Dustan, 1970), it can be regarded as an appropriate beta-adrenergic response to a greater orthostatic shift of blood volume and associated reduction of forward stroke output that is exaggerated in taller and leaner persons. For reasons already discussed, some patients may exhibit an abnormal orthostatic response that leads to an alpha-adrenergically mediated vasoconstriction and increased peripheral resistance that serves to maintain the cardiac output and results in a higher standing than supine blood pressure. The orthostatically induced release of epinephrine stimulates a relatively augmented noradrenergic release that induces vasoconstriction and leads to a reduced 24-hour excretion of sodium that is inversely correlated with that of norepinephrine. It is therefore not unexpected that some subjects with MVP can exhibit a chronic increase of peripheral resistance that is associated with sustained elevation of the blood pressure, in contrast to the usually observed lower blood pressures associated with MVP (Savage et al., 1983; Devereux, Brown, Kramer-Fox, et al., 1982). In comparison with the general population, subjects with MVP thus exhibit less weight for height and lower blood pressure. It might be hypothesized that a taller and leaner individual has a relatively greater orthostatic difficulty maintaining the cardiac output and blood pressure, and exhibits enhanced postural epinephrine release in an attempt to stimulate an increase of noradrenergic activity that can induce compensatory hemodynamic responses. Physical activity induces increased release of epinephrine which serves to enhance LV function and to increase heart rate and systolic blood pressure. A metabolically related vasodilation in the muscular tissues lowers blood pressure and stimulates release of norepinephrine. Such normal responses are increased in the upright position and become exaggerated in those with postural hypotension (Stratton, Pfeiffer, Ritchie, & Halter, 1985). A mechanistic explanation for the occurrence of MVP in tall and lean persons and otherwise in subjects with a narrower antero-posterior diameter is thus consonant with physiological findings.

The somatotypically enhanced beta-adrenergic response to stress and postural changes (Stratton et al., 1985) thus predisposes taller and leaner persons and those with narrower antero-posterior chest diameters to a failure of mitral leaflet coaptation and subsequent valve prolapse. The smaller left ventricular volume and size and enhanced LV contractility engendered by release of epinephrine probably exerts a greater tugging effect on the chordae of such persons because their hearts tend to be suspended more vertically in the thorax and to exhibit a more dynamic systolic contraction, compared to shorter and heavier individuals whose hearts are more horizontally aligned in the thoracic cavity. A mechanistic explanation is also supported by the fact that, in family studies, the prevalence of MVP is the same regardless of the presence or absence of straight backs or pectus in the proband. The observed thoracic skeletal configurations associated with MVP (Salomon et al., 1975) simply result in the same type of narrower antero-posterior chest diameter that is often found in tall, thin subjects.

The age- and sex-dependent expressions in the transmission of MVP (Devereux, Brown, Kramer-Fox, et al., 1982) probably reside in concurrent changes in autonomic structure and function, and these are sex- and age-related. An early age/sex change appears to occur at puberty and is reflected in the experience with blood pressure levels. Blood pressures are similar in male and female children prior to puberty. An increased pressor response to stress occurs in both sexes after puberty but is greater in males. In adolescence, males exhibit higher systolic blood pressures at rest. These differences are probably related to the differential sex hormone effects that occur at puberty (Von Eiff, Gogolin, Jacobs, & Neus, 1985) and probably contribute to the generally lower prevalence of hypertension in females. Although childhood pressure levels track into young adulthood, later blood pressures are best predicted by adolescent rather than early childhood measures (Clarke & Lauer, 1985), confirming the importance of the neuroendocrine changes that occur at puberty.

The sequential response to stress involves an increased release of epinephrine followed by a modest increase of norepinephrine, the magnitude of which is sex-dependent. In general, females appear to have a higher E/NE response ratio compared to males (Frankenhaeuser, 1978), and this underlies their greater beta-adrenergic type of stress response. During adult life age-related decrements occur in the metabolism and content of catecholamines in certain brain and neurotransmitter regions. However, plasma levels of epinephrine remain unchanged with aging, whereas those of norepinephrine tend to increase (Izzo, Smith, Larrabee, & Kallay, 1985), perhaps because of an increased need to maintain cardiovascular responsiveness. It can be hypothesized that a decreased prevalence of MVP in females after their forties results from this age-related increase of noradrenergic response to stress. This in turn diminishes the effects of beta-adrenergic stimulation that favor occurrence of MVP in younger females, particularly in those with somato-typically enhanced response of epinephrine to stressors.

There is a high prevalence of MVP in subjects with anxiety disorder (Dean, 1985; Boudoulas, Reynolds, Mazzaferri, & Wooley, 1980), and this relationship has suggested a common genetic basis. However, the familial risk for anxiety and panic disorders is not dependent on the presence of MVP. Moreover, neither the symptomatic response of patients with panic disorders to lactate infusion nor their prevention by appropriate pretreatment (Gorman, Fyer, Glicklich, King, & Klein, 1981) are dependent on the presence of

MVP. Such findings are among a number of reasons to support a belief that anxiety disorders and MVP often coexist merely because the former is associated with increased beta-adrenergic stimulation rather than considering a common genetic factor that resides in an inherited dysautonomia. Much of the evidence that led to the latter conclusion was based on studies of symptomatic patients. In fact, symptoms occur in well under half of patients with MVP and there may be no differences of anxiety or evidence of autonomic dysfunction in an unselected series of subjects with and without MVP (Chesler, Weir, Braatz, & Francis, 1985). Aside from palpitation, the symptoms associated with MVP are beta-adrenergically mediated, and are causally related to secretion of epinephrine (Nezu et al., 1985), hence are more prevalent in subjects with anxiety disorders.

Anxiety disorders are associated with increased beta-adrenergic stimulation, and higher levels and surges of epinephrine may be partly responsible not only for the symptoms that can occur in patients with MVP (Chesler et al., 1985), but also for symptoms and panic attacks that occur in patients with anxiety disorders (Boudoulas et al., 1983; Rainey et al., 1984). Although anxiety disorders may be related to a genetic deficiency of hormone or neurotransmitter that normally regulates anxiety (Paul & Skolnick, 1981), the locus ceruleus is rich in cells containing norepinephrine and changes in its metabolism may control psychological anxiety, fear, and panic (Uhde et al., 1984). Central catecholamine metabolism is probably involved in the subjective symptoms of anxiety disorders, but far less so for the physiological accompaniments of anxiety. It is thus not surprising that beta-adrenergic blocking agents may be useful for the treatment of symptomatic manifestations of MVP, but do not prevent panic attacks when such disorders coexist. Such considerations lead to the conclusion that idiopathic MVP may sometimes be a marker for anxiety disorders, but does not coexist because of a common genetic defect. In considering the augmented beta-adrenergic stimulation that is observed in patients with anxiety disorders, however, their frequent exhibition of MVP can readily be understood.

Although anxiety disorders may lead to enhanced beta-adrenergic stimulation and in turn be responsible for an associated high prevalence of MVP, the fact that such subjects tend to exhibit lower blood pressures (Devereux, Brown, & Lutas, 1982; Savage et al., 1983) may negate a significant role of emotional anxiety in the pathogenesis of hypertension, despite common beliefs to the contrary. The lower blood pressures associated with MVP may also be responsible for a possible lower rate of coronary artery disease in such persons (Schocken, Worden, Harrison, & Spielberger, 1984; Sprafkin, McCroskery, Lantinga, & Hills, 1984).

Although there is a lack of male penetrance in families with MVP (Devereux, Brown, Kramer-Fox et al., 1982), it is significant that male subjects with idiopathic MVP also appear to exhibit the same somatotypic associations that prevail in females, and that symptomatic MVP is prone to occur in males during periods of increased anxiety, such as in combat soldiers (DaCosta, 1871; MacLean, 1867).

Type A Behavior Pattern and Ischemic Heart Disease

The role of Type A behavior pattern (TABP) in ischemic heart disease (IHD) represents a different relationship of emotions to cardiovascular disease and occurs in contrast to the association of anxiety with various other cardiovascular disorders. As far back as 1892, Osler had linked the increased incidence of IHD in the western world to factors of stress and certain behaviors. However, the concept of TABP did not arise until well into the 20th century when it became apparent that the conventional risk factors did not explain either the historical changes in rate of IHD or their geographic distribution (Rosenman, 1983; Rosenman & Chesney, 1982). The incidence of IHD increased after World War I, primarily in middle-aged males who resided in highly urbanized and densely populated, industrialized areas. This relationship can be observed by comparing rates of IHD mortality in the United States in 1950 with their altered distribution in the early 1970s. During these two decades there had occurred a greatly increased IHD rate in the southeastern region associated with the area's increased industrialization and population densification. It also became apparent that the different rates of IHD that were observed in various European countries could not be ascribed to differences of diet, physical activity, or the conventional risk factors. Nor can the recent decline of IHD mortality in the United States and certain other countries be easily explained by changes in such factors.

The historical changes and geographic differences in incidence of IHD that are unexplained by the classic risk factors promoted a broad search for additional pathogenetic influences, resulting in a separate category of risk factors that are generally related to concepts of stress and to different individual perceptions of the environmental milieu and its stressors. The latter consideration led to the conceptualization of the TABP in the 1950s, along with direct observation of the behavior of relatively younger and middle-aged patients with IHD. If the incidence of IHD is particularly associated with urbanization, population density, and industrialization in the western world, then it is perhaps the associated need for competitiveness that has particularly engendered the TABP in susceptible individuals. This is not an evolutionary development and may therefore be regarded as inappropriately directed (Montagu, 1976). There is good reason to believe that such factors may underlie the constellation of Type A behaviors, which include increased aggressiveness and drive, and in turn lead to an accelerated pace of activities and increased potential for hostility (Rosenman et al., 1964; Rosenman, 1978; Rosenman, 1985)

In the WCGS, the TABP was independently associated with a significantly high incidence of IHD (Rosenman et al., 1976), a finding that was replicated in a number of other prevalent as well as prospective studies conducted in the United States, Europe, and elsewhere (Rosenman & Chesney, 1982). We have recently completed a retrospective analysis of the structured interviews (Rosenman, 1978) given to the WCGS participants at intake into the study (Rosenman et al., 1964), for the purpose of assessing their Type A or B behavior patterns. This new analysis utilized the methodology developed by Hecker to study the various TABP components. He did a blind analysis of the intake interviews that had been given to the 257 subjects who developed IHD during the 9-year follow up, and to two control subjects paired with each IHD case by age and company of employment. It was found (Hecker, Chesney, Black, & Rosenman, in press) that among the component Type A behaviors, strong predictors of IHD were competitiveness, hostility/anger dimensions, and characteristic Type A vocal stylistics (Rosenman, 1978). These findings confirmed an earlier similar type of blind analysis done by Bortner (Matthews, Glass, Rosenman, & Bortner, 1977) that was accomplished with different methodology. The relationship of the hostility component of the TABP to the prevalence and incidence of IHD and to the severity of coronary atherosclerosis was observed in an earlier analysis of WCGS subjects who were excluded from follow up because of silent myocardial infarction (Jenkins, Rosenman, & Friedman, 1966), as well as by a number of other investigators (Rosenman & Chesney, 1982; Rosenman, 1985).

Behavioral stimuli evoke autonomic and associated neurohormonal cardiovascular responses that may accelerate coronary atherosclerosis and precipitate its complications, leading to an increased incidence of IHD. Type A persons exhibit a greater magnitude as well as frequency of such responses in their daily milieu (Rosenman & Chesney, 1982). The drive for preservation of the species and the self leads to a type of competitiveness and aggression that is biologically adaptive, life-serving, and phylogenetically programmed (Montagu, 1976). This type of response is common to both animals and humans, whereas many other forms of aggression are probably not and may therefore be biologically maladaptive. They arise solely out of the human experience because they are exclusively found in human beings. In contrast, as elegantly discussed by Montagu (1976), the principal factor operating in animal evolution is cooperation rather than the divisiveness and the inappropriate aggression, competitiveness, and conflict that characterize the human experience and are exemplified by the coronary-prone facets of the TABP.

TABP is a constellation of behaviors that are used to cope with the human experience. Although TABP does not equate with anxiety, as usually considered, it is possible that there is an underlying anxiety that is associated with a threat of failure that in turn leads to Type A competitiveness, aggressiveness, accelerated pace of activities, and the hostile behaviors that are associated with an increased incidence of IHD (Rosenman, 1983; Rosenman & Chesney 1982; Rosenman, 1985; Rosenman et al., 1976).

References

Baer, P.E., Collins, F.H., Bourenoff, G.C., & Ketchel, M.F. (1979). Assessing personality factors in essential hypertension with a brief self-report instrument. *Psychosomatic Medicine, 16,* 721–730.

Beard, G. (1867). Neurasthenia, or nervous exhaustion? *Boston Medical Surgical Journal, LXXX,* 161–164.

Boudoulas, H., Reynolds, J.C., Mazzaferri, E., & Wooley C.F. (1980). Metabolic studies in mitral valve prolapse syndrome: A neuroendocrine-cardiovascular process. *Circulation, 61,* 1200–1205.

Boudoulas, H., Reynolds, J.C., Mazzaferri, E., & Wooley, C.F. (1983). Mitral valve prolapse syndrome: The effect of adrenergic stimulation. *Journal of the American College of Cardiology, 2,* 638–644.

Brody, M.J., Natelson, B.H., Anderson, E., Folkow, B.U.G., Levy, M.N., Obrist, P.A., Reis, D.F., Rosenman, R.H., Watanabe, A.N., Williams, R.S., & Zipes, D.P. (1987). Behavioral mechanisms in hypertension. *Report of Task Force No.3, American Heart Association Conference on Biobehavioral Medicine and Cardiovascular Disease, Sea Island* (February 3–7, 1985). *Circulation,* Part II, *76:* I-84-88

Brown, M.J. (1985). Hypokalemia from beta-2-receptor stimulation by circulating epinephrine. *American Journal Cardiology, 56,* 3D–9D.

Brown, M.J., Brown, D.C., & Murphy, M.B. (1983). Hypokalemia from beta-2-receptor stimulation by circulating epinephrine. *New England Journal of Medicine, 309,* 1414–1419.

Bruhn, J.G., Paredes, A., Adsett, C.A. et al. (1984). Psychological predictors of sudden death in myocardial infarction. *Journal of Psychosomatic Medicine, 18,* 449–454.

Burchell, H.B. (1984). Letter to editor. *New England Journal of Medicine, 311,* 1520–1521.

Cassem, N.H., & Hackett, T.P. (1977). Psychological aspects of myocardial infarction. *Medical Clinics of North America, 61,* 711–721.

Channick, B.J., Adlin, E.V., Marks, A.D., Denenberg, B.S., Chakko, C.S., & Spann, J.F. (1981). Hyperthyroidism and mitral valve prolapse. *New England Journal of Medicine, 305,* 497–500.

Chesler, E., Weir, E.K., Braatz, G.A., & Francis, G.S. (1985). Normal catecholamine and hemodynamic responses to orthostatic tilt in subjects with mitral valve prolapse: Correlation with psychologic testing. *Journal of the American College of Cardiology, 5,* 504.

Chesney, M.A. (1986). Hypertension: Biobehavioral influences and their implications for treatment. In T.H. Schmidt, T.M. Dembroski, & G. Blumchen (Eds.), *Biological and psychological factors in cardiovascular disease* (pp. 568–583). Heidelberg: Springer-Verlag.

Clarke, W.R., & Lauer, R.M. (1985). Lipids and blood pressure in childhood predict adult risk: The Muscatine Study. *Circulation, 68,* III–451.

Conway, J. (1983). Hemodynamic aspects of essential hypertension in humans. *Physiological Review, 63,* 617–660.

Cottier, C., Shapiro, K., & Julius, S. (1984). Treatment of mild hypertension with progressive muscle relaxing: Predictive value of indexes of sympathetic tone. *Archives of Internal Medicine, 144,* 1954–1958.

Culpepper, W.S. III, Sodt, P.C., Messerli, F.H., Ruschhaupt, D.G., & Arcilla, R.A. (1983). Cardiac status in juvenile borderline hypertension. *Annals of Internal Medicine, 98,* 1–7.

Curatolo, P.W., & Robertson, D. (1983). The health consequences of caffeine. *Annals of Internal Medicine, 98,* 641–653.

DaCosta, J.M. (1871). On irritable heart. *American Journal of Medical Science, 61,* 17–52.

Dean, G.A. (1985). Mitral valve prolapse. *Hospital Practice, September,* 75–82.

Dembroski, D.M., MacDougall, J.M., Cardozo, S.R., & Krug-Fite, J. (1985). Selective cardiovascular effects of stress and cigarette smoking in young women.*Health Psychology, 4*, 153–167.

Devereux, R.B., Brown, W.T., & Lutas, E.M. (1982). Association of mitral valve prolapse with low body weight and low blood pressure. *Lancet, 2*, 792–795.

Devereux, R.B., Brown, W.T., Kramer-Fox, R., & Laragh J.H. (1982). Inheritance of mitral valve prolapse: Effect of age and sex on gene expression. *Annals of Internal Medicine, 97*, 826–832.

Diamond E.L. (1982). The role of anger and hostility in essential hypertension and coronary heart disease. *Psychological Bulletin, 92*, 410–433.

Dyckner, T., Helmers, R., & Wester, P.O. (1984). Cardiac dysrhythmias in patients with acute myocardial infarction. *Acta Medicus Scandinavica, 216*, 127–132.

Elias, M.F., & Streeten, D.H.P. (Eds.). (1980). *Hypertension and cognitive processes.* Mount Desert, ME: Beech-Hill.

Esler, M., Julius, S., Zweiffer, A., Randall, O., Harburg, E., Gardiner, H., & De-Quattro, V. (1977). Mild high-renin essential hypertension: Neurogenic human hypertension? *New England Journal of Medicine, 296*, 405–411.

Falkner, B., Onesti, G., Angelakos, E.T., Fernandez, M., & Langman, C. (1974). Cardiovascular response to mental stress in normal adolescents with hypertensive parents. *Hypertension, 1*, 23–30.

Falkner, B., Onesti, G., & Hamstra, B. (1981). Stress response characteristics of adolescents with high genetic risk for essential hypertension: A five-year follow-up. *Clinical and Experimental Hypertension, 3*, 583–591.

Feldman, T., Borow, K.M., Neumann, A., Sarne, D.H., Land, R.M., & DeGroot, L.J. (1985). What are the factors influencing augmented left ventricular shortening in hyperthyroidism? *Journal of the American College of Cardiology, 5*, 535.

Frankenhaeuser, M. (1978). *Psychoneuroendocrine sex differences in adaption to the psychosocial environment.* New York: Academic Press.

Frankenhaeuser, M. (1982). The sympathetic-adrenal and pituitary-adrenal response to challenge: Comparison between the sexes. In T.M. Dembroski, T.H. Schmidt, & G. Blumchen (Eds.), *Biobehavioral bases of coronary heart disease* (pp. 91–105). Basel, Switzerland: Karger.

Frohlich, E.D., Kozul, V.J., Tarazi, R.C., & Dustan, H.P. (1970). Physiological comparison of labile and essential hypertension. *Circulation Research, 55* (Supplement 1), 26–27.

Gentry, W.D., Balder, L., Oude-Weme, J.D., Musch, F., & Gary, H.E. (1983). Type A/B differences in coping with acute myocardial infarction: Further considerations. *Heart and Lung, 12*, 212–214.

Gorman, J.M., Fyer, A.F., Glicklich, J., King, D.L., & Klein, D.F. (1981). Mitral valve prolapse and panic disorders: Effect of imipramine. In D.F. Klein, & J. Rabkin (Eds.), *Anxiety: New research and changing concepts* (pp. 317–325). New York: Raven Press.

Harvey, W. (1984). Exercitatio de motu cordis et sanguinis. Cited in T.P. Hackett & J.F. Rosenbaum, *Emotion, psychiatric disorders, and the heart* (pp. 1826–1946). In E. Braunwald (Ed.), *Heart Disease.* Philadelphia: Saunders.

Hecker, M.L.H., Chesney, M.A., Black, G.W., & Rosenman, R.H. (in press). A retrospective analysis of coronary-prone Type A behaviors in the Western Collaborative Group Study.

Hennekens, C.H., Lown, B., Rosener, B., Grufferman, S., & Dalen, J. (1980). Ventricular premature beats and coronary risk factors. *American Journal of Epidemiology*, *112*, 93–99.

Henry, J.P., & Stephens, P.M. (1977). *Stress, health, and the social environment.* New York: Springer-Verlag.

Izzo, J.L., Smith, R.J., Larrabee, P.S., & Kallay, M.C. (1985). Plasma norepinephrine, age and vasoconstriction in essential hypertension. *Circulation, 68*, III–295.

Jenkins, C.D., Rosenman, R.H., & Friedman, M.J. (1966). Components of the coronary-prone behavior pattern: Their relation to silent myocardial infarction and blood lipids. *Journal of Chronic Diseases, 19*, 599–605.

Jenkins, C.D., Stanton, B.A., Klein, M.D., Savageau, J.A., & Harken, D.E. (1983). Correlates of angina pectoris among men awaiting coronary by-pass surgery. *Psychosomatic Medicine, 45*, 141–153.

Jennings, J.R., & Follansbee, W.P. (1984). Type A and ectopy in patients with coronary artery disease and controls. *Journal of Psychosomatic Research, 28*, 449–454.

Klatsky, A.L., Friedman, G.D., Siegelaum, A.B., & Gerad, M.J. (1977). Alcohol consumption and blood pressure. *New England Journal of Medicine, 296*, 1194–1200.

Krakoff, L.R., Dziedzic, S., Mann, S.J., Felton, K., & Yeager, K. (1985). Plasma epinephrine concentrations in healthy men: Correlation with systolic blood pressure and rate-pressure product. *Journal of the American College of Cardiology, 5*, 352.

Lader, M. (1984). Neurotransmitters and anxiety: Overview. *Psychopathology, 17*, 3–7.

Lown, B. (1979). Sudden cardiac death: The major challenge confronting contemporary cardiology. *American Journal of Cardiology, 43*, 313–328.

Lown, B., & Verrier, R.L. (1976). Neural activity and ventricular fibrillation. *New England Journal of Medicine, 294*, 1165–1170.

MacLean, W.C. (1867). Disease of the heart in the British Army: The cause and the remedy. *British Medical Journal, 1*, 161–164.

Marmot, M.G. (1984). Alcohol and coronary heart disease. *International Journal of Epidemiology, 13*, 160–167.

Matthews, K.A., Glass, D.C., Rosenman, R.H., & Bortner, R.W. (1977). Competitive drive, pattern A and coronary heart disease: A further analysis of some data from the Western Collaborative Group Study. *Journal of Chronic Diseases, 30*, 489–498.

Montagu, A. (1976). *The nature of human aggression.* New York: Oxford University Press.

Neff, J.A. (1984). The stress-buffering role of alcohol consumption: The importance of symptom dimension. *Journal of Human Stress, 10*, 35–42.

Nezu, M., Miura, Y., Adachi, M., Adachi, M., Kimura, S., Toriyabe, S., Ishizuka, Y., Ohashi, H., Sugawara, T., Takahashi, M., Noshiro, T., & Yoshinaga, K. (1985). The effects of epinephrine release in essential hypertension. *Hypertension, 7*, 187–195.

Nixon, P.G.F. (1982). Are there clinically significant prodromal signs and symptoms of impending sudden death? *Practical Cardiology, 8*, 173–183.

Nordrehaug, J.E. (1985). Malignant arrhythmias in relation to serum potassium in acute myocardial infarction. *American Journal of Cardiology, 56*, 20D–23D.

Osler, W. (1892). The Lumelian lectures on angina pectoris. *Lancet, 1*, 829–844.

Paul, S.M., & Skolnick, P. (1981). Benzodiazepine receptors and psychopathological states: Towards a neurobiology of anxiety. In D.F. Klein & J. Rabkin (Eds.), *Anxiety: New research and changing concepts.* New York: Raven Press.

Pickering, T.G., Harshfield, G.A., Kleinert, H.D., Blank, S.B., & Laragh, J.H.

(1982). Blood pressure during normal daily activities, sleep, and exercise: Comparison of values in normal and hypertensive subjects. *Journal of the American Medical Association, 247,* 992–996.

Rainey, M., Ettedgui, R., Pohl, B., Balon, R., Weinberg, P., Yelonek, S., & Berchou, R. (1984). The beta-receptor: Isoproterenol anxiety states. *Psychopathology, 17* (Supplement 3), 40–51.

Reich, P., deSilva, R.A., Lown, B., & Murawski, J. (1981). Acute psychological disturbances preceding life-threatening ventricular arrhythmias. *Journal of the American Medical Association, 246,* 233–235.

Robertson, D., Frolich, J.C., Carr, R.K., Watson, J.T., Hollifield, J.W., Shand, D.E., & Oates, J.A. (1978). Effects of caffeine on plasma renin activity, catecholamines and blood pressure. *New England Journal of Medicine, 298,* 181–186.

Rosenman, R.H. (1978). The interview method of assessment of the coronary-prone behavior pattern. In T.M. Dembroski, S.M. Weiss, J.L. Shields, S.G. Haynes, & M. Feinleib (Eds.), *Coronary-prone behavior* (pp. 55–69). New York: Springer-Verlag.

Rosenman, R.H. (1983). Coronary-prone behavior pattern and coronary heart disease: Implications for the use of beta-blockers in primary prevention. In R.H. Rosenman (Ed.), *Psychosomatic risk factors and coronary heart disease. Indications for specific preventive therapy* (pp. 9–14). Bern: Huber.

Rosenman, R.H. (1985). Health consequences of anger and implications for treatment. In M.A. Chesney & R.H. Rosenman (Eds.), *Anger and hostility in cardiovascular and behavioral disorders* (pp. 103–125). New York: Hemisphere/McGraw-Hill.

Rosenman, R.H., Brand, R.J. Sholtz, R.I., & Friedman, M. (1976). Multivariate prediction of coronary heart disease during 8.5 year follow-up in the Western Collaborative Group Study. *American Journal of Cardiology, 37,* 903–910.

Rosenman, R.H., & Chesney, M.A. (1982). Stress, Type A behavior, and coronary disease. In L. Goldberger & S. Breznitz (Eds.), *Handbook of stress: Theoretical and clinical aspects* (pp. 547–565). New York: Free Press.

Rosenman, R.H., Friedman, M., Straus, R., Jenkins, C.D., Zyzanski, S.J., & Wurm, M. (1964). A predictive study of coronary heart disease: The Western Collaborative Group Study. *Journal of the American Medical Association, 189,* 15–22.

Ruberman, W., Weinblatt, E., & Goldberg, J.D. (1984). Psychosocial influences on mortality after myocardial infarction. *New England Journal of Medicine, 311,* 552–559.

Salmond, C.E., Joseph, J.G., Prior, I.A.M., Stanley, D.G., & Wessen, A.F. (1985). Longitudinal analysis of the relationship between blood pressure and migration: The Tokelau Island migrant study. *American Journal of Epidemiology, 122,* 291–301.

Salomon, J., Shah, P.M., & Heinle, R.A. (1975). Thoracic skeletal abnormalities in mitral valve prolapse. *American Journal of Cardiology, 36,* 32–36.

Savage, D.D., Devereux, R.B., Garrison, R.J., Castelli, W.P., Anderson, J.J., Levy, D., Thomas, H.E., Kannel, W.B., & Feinleib, M. (1983). Mitral valve prolapse in the general population. 2. Clinical features: The Framingham Study. *American Heart Journal, 106,* 577–581.

Schatzkin, A., Cupples, L.A., Neeren, T., Morelock, S., & Kannel, W.B. (1984). Sudden death in the Framingham Heart Study. *American Journal of Epidemiology, 120,* 889–899.

Schocken, D.D., Worden, T.J., Harrison, E.E., & Spielberger, C.D. (1984). Anxiety differences in patients with angina pectoris, non-anginal chest pain, and coronary artery disease. *Circulation, 70,* 1587.

Schwartz, G.E., Weinberger, D.A., & Singer, J.A. (1981). Cardiovascular differentiation of happiness, sadness, anger and fear following imagery and exercise. *Psychosomatic Medicine, 43*, 343–364.

Schwartz, P.J. (1984). Stress and sudden cardiac death: The role of the autonomic nervous system. *Journal of Psychology, 2*, 7–13.

Shekelle, R.B., Schoenberger, J.A., & Stamler, J. (1976). Correlates of the JAS Type A behavior score. *Journal of Chronic Diseases, 29*, 381–394.

Skinner, J.E. (1985). Psychosocial stress and sudden cardiac death: Brain mechanisms. In R.E. Beamish, P.K. Singal, & N.A. Dhalla (Eds.), *Stress and heart disease* (pp. 44–59). Boston: Martinus Nijhoff Publishers.

Skinner, J.E., Lie, J.T., & Entman, M.L. (1975). Modification of ventricular fibrillation latency following coronary artery occlusion in the conscious pig: The effects of psychological stress and beta-adrenergic blockade. *Circulation, 51*, 656–667.

Skinner, J.E., & Reed, J.C. (1981). Blockade of frontocortical-brainstem pathway prevents ventricular fibrillation of the ischemic heart in pigs. *American Journal of Physiology, 240*, H156–163.

Sprafkin, R.P., McCroskery, J.H., Lantinga, L.J., & Hills, N. (1984). Cardiovascular and psychological characteristics of patients with chest pain. *Behavioral Medicine Update, 6*, 11.

Strahlendorf, J., & Strahlendorf, H. (1981). Response of locus coeruleus neurons to direct application of ethanol. *Society of Neuroscience Abstracts, 104*, 7B.

Stratton, J.R., Pfeiffer, M.A., Ritchie, J.L., & Halter, J.B. (1985). Hemodynamic effects of epinephrine: Concentration effect study in humans. *Journal of Applied Physiology, 58*, 1199–1206.

Taggart, P., Carruthers, M., & Somerville, W. (1973). Electrocardiograms, plasma catecholamines, and lipids, and their modification by exprenolol when speaking before an audience. *Lancet, 2*, 341–346.

Talbott, E., Kuller, L.H., & Perper, J. (1981). Sudden unexpected death in women: Biologic and psychosocial origins. *American Journal of Epidemiology, 144*, 671–682.

Trimarco, B., Ricciardelli, B., De Luca, N., De Simone, A., Cuocolo, A., Galva, M.D., Picotti, G.B., & Condorelli, M. (1985). Participation of endogenous catecholamines in the regulation of left ventricular mass in progeny of hypertensive patients. *Circulation, 72*, 38–46.

Uhde, T.W., Boulenger, J.P., Post, R.M., Siever, L.J., Vittone, B.J., Jimerson, D.C., & Roy-Berne, P.P. (1984). Fear and anxiety: Relationship to noradrenergic function. *Psychopathology, 17* (Supplement 3), 8–23.

Von Eiff, A.W., Gogolin, E., Jacobs, U., & Neus, H. (1985). Sex specific blood pressure regulation before and after puberty. *Journal of Hypertension, 3*, 416.

Vuori, I., Makarainen, M., & Jaaskelainen, A. (1978). Sudden death and physical activity. *Cardiology, 63*, 287–304.

Weiss, K.J., & Rosenberg, D.J. (1985). Prevalence of anxiety disorder among alcoholics. *Journal of Clinical Psychology, 46*, 3–5.

Williams, J.C. (1836). *Practical observations on nervous and sympathetic palpitation of the heart.* London: Longman, Rees, Orme, Browne.

2

Hassles, Health, and Happiness

Norman S. Endler

In this chapter Endler surveys the history of attitudes toward *mental illness*, particularly from the perspective of the effects of stress upon health. We are provided with an analysis of the varying concepts of stress itself, as well as a discussion of the relationships among stress, anxiety, vulnerability, and illness. These reviews give us a deft sequel to those presented in the previous chapter. The theme of differences in vulnerability of individuals to the effects of stress and anxiety complements Rosenman's preceding discussion of the multiplicity of factors involved in cardiovascular health and illness. Endler's unique interactional approach to the study of anxiety, and indeed personality, is given full exposition here, with particular emphasis upon his most recent investigations. The research upon a myriad of variables, as they are related to stress and coping, is detailed here; in addition to stress, anxiety, and vulnerability, the relationship of these variables to such factors as biochemical changes, cognitive factors, hassles, illness, stressful life events, and the Type A behavior pattern are all reviewed. This is presented in the context of dynamic interactionism, with special emphases upon three approaches: the interaction model of personality, the multidimensional interaction model of anxiety, and the dynamic interaction stress model. Before concluding the chapter, Endler gives emphasis to the roles of optimism, self-efficacy, and perceived control in stressful situations in determining health and happiness. The interaction theme continues with his conclusion that there are dynamic and complex relationships among stress, anxiety, vulnerability, and coping, a fact amply demonstrated by his impressive review of the literature.

—EDITOR

The relationship between stress and illness has a short history, but a long past. Stress, especially those aspects encapsulated in our daily life experiences, has been perceived as a causal factor in both physical and mental illness. According to Lief (1948), Adolph Meyer was one of the first individuals to assess the effects of daily life experiences on consequent illness. Meyer (see Lief, 1948) in his psychobiological theories, noted that in examining life problems, one must focus on the *interaction* of an individual organism with life situations, and be concerned with the mind-body relationship. The investigation of this relationship is not new, and the debate whether mind and body should be considered as parallel systems or as interacting with one another, within the same system, goes back at least to the Stone Age.

Attitudes Toward Mental Health

The notion of demonology, that is the belief that an evil being such as the devil could reside within a person and take control of the mind, although prominent in the Middle Ages, actually originated in the Stone Age. The ancient Hebrews, during the time of Jesus Christ, believed that behavior was controlled by good or evil spirits that had taken possession of the person (Endler, 1982). Demonological beliefs and values were not unique to the early Christians and Hebrews, but also pervaded the thoughts of the ancient Chinese, Egyptians, and Greeks. "These demons were treated by flogging and starvation and by more benign methods, such as ritual prayers, loud noises, and coercion of the person possessed to drink terrible-tasting brews. Deviant behaviour was often treated with exorcism" (Endler, 1982, p.133). Hippocrates, however, accepted the somatogenic hypothesis about mental illness, and suggested such treatments as quietness, sobriety, sexual abstinence, and care in selecting drink and food. He believed that this treatment was healthy for both the body and the brain.

After the death of Galen (who also accepted the somatogenic hypothesis) in the third century AD, the Dark Ages for the treatment and study of mental illness began. There were few subsequent advances in medicine and Roman physicians believed in superstitious explanations of illness and in demonology. However, with the advent of Christianity, being possessed by evil spirits was considered an insult to both God and the Church. "Therefore the person who was mentally ill was doubly cursed—first by being ill and secondly by antagonizing the church" (Endler, 1982, p.134). Medical practice was heavily influenced by religious factors, and many of the healing functions of the physician were absorbed by the priest.

During the Middle Ages, priests had the prime responsibility for the treatment of mental illness. They prayed for the ill and sprinkled them with holy water. The priests became zealous in their attempts to rid the patients of the spirit of Satan, and cursed both Satan and the patient, eventually substituting torture for prayer as a means of punishing the devil within the patient.

The religious establishment focused on two types of possession by the devil. In one set of instances the patient was involuntarily seized by the devil as God's punishment for committed sins—a personal misfortune. In other instances, the priests believed that persons intentionally became involved with a contract with the devil and became witches with supernatural powers, working at the devil's bidding. In this case the witches would sicken cattle, strike down their enemies, ruin crops, influence the weather, ruin the community, and make men impotent. Commencing in the 16th century the distinction between these two forms of possession by the devil became fuzzy and many innocent people were labeled as witches or heretics and held responsible for causing floods and pestilence (Endler, 1982).

During the 14th century, the insane were perceived as being dangerous and therefore became the targets of persecution. Ironically, the physical care for the insane was better in the Middle Ages than in the 17th and 18th centuries. When Bethlehem Hospital in London (later called "Bedlam") was originally opened, the inmates were treated with concern and compassion. Furthermore, when the patients were well enough to leave the hospital under the supervision of their relatives, they were given badges that would readmit them to the hospital if they became sick again. The social support of the community was so sympathetic and attentive that vagrants often counterfeited the badges in order to be considered ex-patients of Bethleham.

Not everything was doom and gloom, however. One source of enlightenment was Johann Weyer, a 16th-century German physician, born in 1515 in Grave, on the Meuse in Holland. Weyer contended that most "witches" were physically or mentally ill, and that "witch-hunting" was unjust and unconscionable. He was probably the founder of modern psychiatry, and the first to specialize in mental illness. His aim was to demonstrate that "witches" were mentally ill and should thus be treated by physicians and not by the clergy.

Weyer studied the absurdities of witchcraft for 12 years and in 1563 he published his important book *De Praestigiis Daemonum* (The Deception of Demons), a point-by-point rebuttal of *Malleus Maleficarum* (The Witches' Hammer). He believed that the illnesses that were attributed to being a witch and being possessed by the devil came from natural causes. He tried to prove that mental illnesses were neither sacred nor supernatural. However, he was criticized by his Renaissance contemporaries (see Endler, 1982).

The Renaissance was a transition point for shifting Western civilization's orientation from superstition to reality. The goal was to determine the truth about man on scientific, philosophical, artistic, and political grounds. Objective observation was used to learn more about human minds and bodies. Both the 17th and 18th centuries constituted an age of objective observation and of reason. The Royal Academy of Science (now the Royal Society) was founded in London in 1662; the Academie Royale des Sciences in Paris in 1666. Scientists during the period included Boyle, Descartes, Galileo, Harvey, Kepler, Newton, and Pascal.

In the field of mental health, Robert Burton, a clergyman, published *The Anatomy of Melancholy* in 1621 and there were five subsequent editions in 30 years. This book, a classic in the field, is a medical treatise on melancholy, which discusses etiology, symptoms, and cures as they were known in the 17th century.

As a result of the explosion of medical and scientific knowledge during the 17th and 18th centuries, it became necessary to synthesize, integrate, and systematize all the new information. Unfortunately, the scientific and medical orientation to mental illness did not automatically lead to a more humane treatment of the insane. The categorization of the symptoms of the mentally ill was thwarted by the fact that clinicians had few opportunities to observe patients directly; this made it difficult to classify patients.

By 1800 physicians had reported and systematically classified their observations. Psychiatric classification by prominent clinicians such as Philippe Pinel (1745–1826) and Vincenzo Chiarugi (1759–1820) produced a general nosology, but alas, no basic understanding of emotional problems. Classification without a psychological understanding of mental illness is not of much use because it does not lead to explanation.

Unfortunately, classification can become ossified, an end to itself, and be influenced by political and social factors. This was true of the earliest attempts at classification. The present DSM-III classification scheme is also influenced by social and political factors. At the end of the 18th century, treatment involving primitive physiological and psychological methods was based primarily on speculation, rather than being derived from the classification schemes of that era.

Herman Boerhaave (1668–1738), a Dutch physician, was influenced by Hippocrates and based his classification on the new discredited idea of the relationship between illness and the four body humors. "Psychotherapy" included bloodletting, purgatives, and dousing patients with ice cold water.

Philippe Pinel (1745–1826) proposed a classification scheme of mental illness late in the 18th century. He categorized the psychoses into manias without delirium, manias with delirium, melancholia, and dementia, on the basis of systematic descriptions of symptoms. Pinel focused on problems of attention, memory, and judgment and emphasized the importance of the emotions in mental illness. He believed that mental illness was due to a lesion in the central nervous system; the somatogenic hypothesis. Pinel postulated that mental illness was a natural phenomenon and a function of heredity and *life events*, including emotional experience. In addition he was concerned with social reform. His methods constituted the first of three major advances in the treatment of mental illness.

Although mentally ill persons had not been tortured at the stake for some time, their position during the Enlightenment, the 18th century, was not completely pleasant. Mentally ill persons who were not hospitalized frequently wandered through the countryside, and were scorned, ridiculed, and sometimes beaten.

There are a number of reasons why patients were treated so harshly during the Enlightenment. First, there was almost complete ignorance about the causes of mental illness. There was progress being made about understanding physical illness. Second, at that time it was believed that mental illness was incurable. Third was the fear or dread of the insane; a fear of the deviant and unknown (see Alexander & Selesnick, 1966).

Although there is still a stigma attached to mental illness (see Endler, 1982), remarkable progress with respect to psychotherapy and somatotherapy has occcured within the last century. In general, there have been three major advances in the treatment of mental illness, two of them within the last 90 years. The first advance was the unshackling of the inmates in the asylums in the 1790s. The second one was the advent of psychoanalysis as formulated by Sigmund Freud, about 1900, and the third one was the biochemical revolution in the 1950s.

The reasons we have devoted so much time to discussing the historical antecedents of attitudes towards mental illness is to provide a historical context for understanding present day attitudes and to demonstrate that negative attitudes are not unique to our era. Let us now discuss some of the early work on life changes and ill health, that is, the effects of stress on physical and mental health.

Stress, Anxiety, Vulnerability, and Illness

As mentioned earlier, many advances have been made in the technology of medicine from the Renaissance to the present. Because of the advances in medicine and medical technology, physicians focused on the body rather than on the mind, whereas philosophers and theologians focused on the mind. For about a 300-year period, physical evidence (e.g., organic and cellular changes) and pathology were the prime basis for the assessment and treatment of illness. Today, however, the focus has changed and we are aware that physical health and illness are dynamically interactive with the social and psychological environment (see Taylor, 1986). Instead of treating mind and body as dual entities, the present focus is on the interaction of mind and body with respect to health and illness. Not only is it believed that physical exercise reduces stress and "inoculates" us against illness, but also that relaxation and psychological well-being promotes good physical health.

Stress

Most of us are aware of the effects that stress has on our physical and psychological well-being. The concept of stress as used in physiology and psychology is borrowed from the field of physics. In physics, stress, was first used to indicate a mechanical force acting on a body, with strain being the reaction to stress (Harris & Levey, 1975). One of the earliest contributions to stress research in the life sciences was the work conducted by Walter B. Cannon

(1932) on the fight-flight response, which indicated that this response is adaptive because it permits the organism to respond rapidly to threat. When a threat is perceived, the body is quickly aroused and motivated. There is increased action in the autonomic nervous system and the endocrine system. While the fight-flight response is adaptive, it can also be harmful to the person, because it disrupts physiological and emotional functioning. When both fight or flight are not possible, the exposure to continued stress may cause physiological damage and illness.

Mahl (1952) found that prolonged and continuous involvement in anxiety-provoking situations leads to excessive secretion of hydrochloric acid, and in some cases, ulcers. Wolf and Wolff (1947) conducted similar research with both animals and humans and decided that individuals develop distinctive physiological responses that are present in a number of stressful situations. If the physiological pattern is overused (e.g., gastric secretion), then a particular illness may develop (e.g., ulcers). Wolf and Wolff believed that there may be inherited predispositions to respond in a specific physiological manner. Some persons may develop high blood pressure, while others may develop ulcers.

To sum up, situations that are threatening or stressful induce physiological arousal. The arousal is adaptive because it mobilizes a fight or flight reaction. However, this mobilization can also produce illness when there is continuous stress; some people may literally "eat their hearts out." There may be wear and tear on a specific physiological system as a result of continuous stress, especially if there is a genetic predisposition with respect to weakness in a specific organ system.

Probably the most important early work on stress research and theory in the life sciences was that of Hans Selye who published his first article in this area on July 4, 1936 in *Nature* (see Selye, 1956). Since then the stress concept has become a very strong focus of theory, research and treatment (see Appley & Trumbull, 1967; Endler & Edwards, in press; Lazarus & Folkman, 1984; Meichenbaum, 1983). Stress has become a general rubric term, with many related concepts encompassed under the contruct of stress. Appley and Trumbull (1967) have stated:

> Since the term gained some attention, and apparently some status as a research topic, it has been used as a substitute for what might otherwise have been called anxiety, conflict, emotional distress, extreme environmental conditions, ego threat, frustration, threat to security, tension arousal or by some other previously respectable terms (p. 1).

Selye's early work (1956, 1976) on the general adaptation syndrome (GAS) is especially important. This stress syndrome, according to Selye, develops in three stages: (1) the alarm reaction; (2) the stage of resistance; and (3) the stage of exhaustion. According to Selye, stress, in its medical sense is basically the state of wear and tear on the body. The nervous system and the endocrine system are important in maintaining resistance during stress. The concept of stress overlaps with that of anxiety and the two terms have often been used interchangeably. Stress, like the anxiety concept, has been defined in a variety of ways. Selye (1956) focused on physiological responses, and defined stress as a "...*non specific response of the body to any demand*" (Selye, 1976, p. 472).

Lazarus (1976) suggested that "...stress occurs when there are demands on the person which tax or exceed his adjustive resources" (p. 47). Lazarus (1976) has differentiated *physical stressors* (environmental conditions) such as extreme heat or cold and *physical injuries*, from *psychosocial stressors* such as social conditions that may be damaging to the self. Nevertheless, Lazarus (1976) is also cognizant of personality factors and reactions factors that are relevant to stress. Earlier, Lazarus (1966) stated that "we must identify the external and internal forces or stimulus conditions of stress reactions and the intervening structures and processes that determine when and in what form the stress reactions will occur" (p. 134). Stress is obviously a complex construct.

The complexity of the stress construct is discussed by Lazarus (1966) who states that, "The important role of personality factors in producing stress reactions requires that we define stress in terms of transactions between individuals and situations, rather than of either one in isolation" (p. 5). Selye (1976), Lazarus (1966), and Lazarus and Folkman (1984) all conceptualize *stress* as a generic term. Stress refers to "the whole area of problems that includes the stimuli producing stress reactions, the reactions themselves, and the various intervening processes" (Lazarus, 1966, p. 27).

Spielberger (1976) states that historically the stress contruct has referred to both stressors (dangerous stimulus conditions) that elicit anxiety reactions, and the stress reactions themselves (cognitive, affective, behavioral, and physiological changes) that are elicited by stressful stimuli. Both research and theory according to Spielberger (1972) suggest that the concepts of stress and threat could be used to indicate different temporal phases of a process that leads to the evocation of an anxiety reaction. Spielberger (1976) suggests that the term *stress* should denote the *objective* stimulus properties of a situation, and the term *threat* should refer to a person's perception of a situation as danger for that person. Most frequently, situations that are objectively stressful (e.g., earthquakes, loss of one's job) will be perceived as threatening. Nevertheless, "...a stressful situation may not be perceived as threatening by an individual who either does not recognize the inherent danger, or has the necessary skills and experience to cope with it" (Spielberger, 1976, p. 5).

On the other hand, an objectively nonstressful situation may be perceived as dangerous by persons who appraise it as threatening for them. There are a number of factors that determine whether or not a situation is perceived as personally threatening. These factors include the general mood of the person, the objective stimulus cues of the situation, the individual's past experience with related situations, cognitions and memories triggered by the current situation, coping skills, and unconscious factors.

A major consequence of the perception of a situation as threatening (independent of whether or not the situation is objectively stressful) is an elevation in the level of state anxiety. Lazarus (1976) conceptualizes anxiety as a stress emotion, in distinction to positive tone emotions such as love, joy, and exhilaration. Other stress emotions include anger, depression, guilt, and jealousy. According to Lazarus (1976) stress emotions include three main components: subjective or experienced affect, action or impulse to act, and physiological changes. We would add a fourth component, namely cognition.

Anxiety

Anxiety has been a major construct in most theories of personality and abnormal psychology extending from the writings of Freud (1933) to those of cognitive social learning theorists and interactionists (Bandura, 1982, 1986; Edwards & Endler, 1983; Endler, 1978, 1983). Freud focused on anxiety and conflict in the origin of the neuroses. His neurotic process theories had a profound impact on the nomenclature and classification systems relevant to psychological disorders involving anxiety (Millon, 1984). This impact, however, has been diminished in the present classification system of the Diagnostic and Statistical Manual III (DSM III, APA, 1980).

The DSM III (APA, 1980) aimed to minimize theory and to maximize descriptive criteria in the current classification scheme. The "anxiety disorders" class is the major category for psychological disorders in which anxiety is the major feature of the disturbance. Anxiety disorders include phobic disorders, anxiety states, and post-traumatic stress disorders, each of which are further subclassified. About 2% to 4% of the general population may, at some time in their lives, suffer from an anxiety disorder (APA, 1980). This would only include those actively seeking treatment, as there may be others who suffer from anxiety disorders who never seek professional help.

An anxiety disorder, or clinical anxiety, is but a small fraction of what we usually include when we discuss the term anxiety. Anxiety has, at various times, been defined as a stimulus, a response, a drive, a motive, and a trait. May (1950), in referring to our era as "the age of anxiety," points out that in the 1940s it was difficult for psychologists to accept the concept of *normal* anxiety. Although Freud (1920) had earlier emphasized the importance of the construct of anxiety with respect to the neuroses, it was not until the 1950s that "the concept of 'normal' anxiety gradually became accepted in the psychiatric literature" (May, 1969, p. 25).

According to Rollo May (1969), "The poet W. H. Auden published *Age of Anxiety* in 1947, and just after that Bernstein wrote his symphony on that theme. Camus was then writing (1947) about this 'century of fear' and Kafka already had created powerful vignettes of the coming age of anxiety in his novels, most of them as yet untranslated" (p. 25). Today it is commonplace among professionals, artists, and laymen to consider anxiety an important and natural construct that pervades all of our lives. Literally thousands and thousands of articles and books have been published on anxiety since the 1950s. Researchers continue to be concerned about anxiety and its contribution to physical and mental health (see Endler & Edwards, in press). Furthermore, many investigators and practitioners have been concerned with the effects of anxiety on the productivity and well-being of members of society (see Sturgis, 1984).

There have been many diverse attempts at comprehensive theories, various measuring scales, and different methodological formulations with respect to the anxiety concept. Many of these scientific attempts have shed more heat than light. In fact the title of a paper by Lewis (1970) on this construct is "The Ambiguous Word 'Anxiety'."

Lewis (1970) defined anxiety ". . . as an emotional state, with the subjectively experienced quality of fear or a closely related emotion (terror, horror, alarm, fright, panic, trepidation, dread, scare)" (p. 77). He points out that the emotion is unpleasant and directed toward the future, is out of proportion to the threat, and involves subjective and manifest bodily disturbances.

Anxiety is a very complex concept. Endler, Hunt, and Rosenstein (1962), in their "S-R Inventory of Anxiousness," which separates *stimulus situation* from *response* in its format, suggest that a *trait* (concept) such as anxiousness can be conceptualized in at least seven ways: (1) in the *proportion* of situations in which persons exhibit the class of anxiety responses; (2) in the *kinds* of situations in which they exhibit these responses; (3) in the *number of different responses* within the anxiety construct; (4) in the prevalence of various subclasses of responses; (5) in the exhibited *intensity* of the *responses* observed; (6) in the *duration* of the *responses* observed; and (7) in the *relative provocativeness* of the *situations*.

Another important distinction for the anxiety construct is the conceptual distinction between state and trait anxiety. Cicero, before the Christian era, made a basic distinction between *angor* and *anxietas*. "*Angor* is transitory, an outburst; *anxiety* is an abiding predisposition" (Cicero as quoted in Lewis, 1970, p. 62). Endler and Magnusson (1976a) point out the the distinction between state anxiety (A-state), a transitory and emotional condition, and chronic or trait anxiety (A-trait), a relatively stable personality characteristic, is a fundamental one. Spielberger (1972) believed that the conceptual and empirical confusion in anxiety research derives from a failure to differentiate between A-state and A-trait. According to Spielberger (1972) state anxiety is a reaction "consisting of unpleasant consciously perceived feelings of tension and apprehension, with associated activation or arousal of autonomic nervous system" (p. 29). Trait anxiety "refers to relatively stable individual differences in anxiety proneness" (Spielberger, 1975, p. 137).

Vulnerability

There are individual differences in responses to stress and individual differences in anxiety. The term vulnerability is used to refer to the individual differences in susceptability to stressors (cf. Endler & Edwards, in press; Garmezy, 1981). Vulnerability is a function of previous stressors, previous experience (learning), constitutional factors, and genetic (hereditary) factors.

The interaction model of personality proposes that person variables interact with specific environments or situations to affect behavior. This model suggests that a variety of individual differences may be involved in determining a person's vulnerability to specific kinds or intensities of stressors. Individual differences may be emotional, motivational, experiential, or cognitive (Endler, 1983), and may be due to both genetic factors (cf. Singer, 1984) and to learning factors, in interaction with a person's environment (cf. Chess, Thomas, & Birch, 1976).

Dynamic Interactionism

The Interaction Model of Personality

Personality theory and research in general, and research and theory on stress and anxiety specifically, have been influenced by four models: the trait model, the psychodynamic model, the situationism model, and the interaction model (Endler & Magnusson, 1976b, 1976c).

The trait model focuses on interactional factors as determinants of behavior and predicts *relative* consistency in reactions across a wide variety of situations. Trait approaches to anxiety and stress focus on individual differences with respect to predispositions and are concerned with an assessment of these differences (cf. Cattell & Scheier, 1961). The *psychodynamic models* also focus on internal determinants of behavior, such as conflicts, drives, impulses, and motives. Freud's (1933) later theory of anxiety discusses the role of unconscious conflicts between impulses, as well as conflicts between the expression of repressed impulses and internalized societal demands. On the other hand, the *situationism models* emphasize external factors as determinants of behavior (e.g., Dollard & Miller, 1950). Criticisms of these earlier models have been discussed by Endler and Magnusson (1976c) and Endler (1983) who present an *interaction* model of personality. This model, which has empirical support, indicates that the person by situation interaction is an important determinant of behavior.

The interaction model of personality (Endler, 1983) presents a conceptualization for examining the reciprocal influences of persons, situations, and reactions. Situations and persons interact in a dynamic ongoing process, and both kinds of variables affect the perception or meaning of the situation and the reactions to that situation. This model also postulates that the person is an active, intentional agent in the process, and that with respect to person factors, cognitive, motivational, and emotional variables are important. The appraisal, or psychological meaning of the situation for the person, is an essential determining factor for behavior.

There are two methodological models of interactionism: mechanistic and dynamic (Endler & Edwards, 1978; Olweus, 1977; Overton & Reese, 1973). the *mechanistic* model focuses on the interaction of two independent variables in affecting behavior (e.g., the interaction of trait anxiety and situation stress in determining increases in levels of state anxiety). The *dynamic* model focuses on reciprocal causality and the *process* (change) of interaction. Individuals not only respond to situations, but also select, alter, and interpret those situations in which they interact, and are in turn altered by them (Endler, 1983; Lazarus & Folkman, 1984).

A dynamic interaction stress model emphasizes the sequence of the stress process and delineates variable for analysis that are relevant to this interaction process (e.g., appraisal of the stressful situation, coping variables, person, situation, and outcome variables).

The Multidimensional Interaction Model of Anxiety

Endler (1975, 1980, 1983) and Endler, Edwards, and Vitelli, (1985, in press) have proposed a multidimensional interaction model of anxiety. This theoretical model has received wide empirical support in both field and laboratory studies. Three conceptual distinctions are essential to this interaction model: (1) the distinction between trait and state anxiety; (2) the multidimensionality of both trait and state anxiety; and (3) the interaction of congruent dimensions of trait anxiety and situational stress in effecting changes in state anxiety.

Endler's (1975, 1980) interaction model postulates that trait anxiety is multidimensional. Persons differ in anxiety proneness with respect to various dimensions of situations; namely social evaluation threat, physical danger threat, ambiguous threat situations, as well as daily routines (innocuous). Both the specific facet or dimension of trait anxiety and the type or category of threat in a stressful situation must be taken into account in predicting state anxiety responses. Person (P) by Situation (S) interactions leading to change in state anxiety are predicted only when the dimension (or facet) of trait anxiety and the type of situational stress are congruent. This means that a person high on social evaluation trait anxiety will manifest an increase in state anxiety when encountering a social evaluation stress situation (e.g., an exam), but not when encountering a physical danger situation. Figure 2.1 presents a schematic overview of a interaction model of anxiety, stress, and coping.

The Dynamic Interaction Stress Model

Lazarus and Folkman (1984) discuss psychological stress in terms of a person's cognitive appraisal of a specific situation as taxing or exceeding that person's coping resources. In this interactional process model, cognitive appraisal is the "person's continually re-evaluated judgements about de-

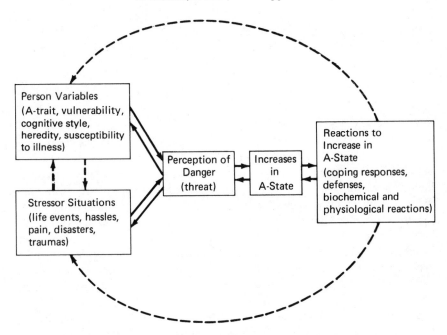

Figure 2.1. Interaction model of anxiety, stress, and coping.

mands and constraints in ongoing transactions with the environment and his or her resources for managing them" (Coyne & Lazarus, 1980, p. 150). Appraisal process influences stress reactions, coping responses, emotions, and adaptational outcomes.

The appraisals process has three phases, namely primary cognitive appraisal, secondary cognitive appraisal, and reappraisal. Primary cognitive appraisal is the evaluation of a situation on the basis of its importance for a person's well-being. Secondary reappraisal is concerned with the person's judgments with respect to available coping resources, options, and constraints, and influences the person's coping responses. Reappraisal involves the process of change in judgments about the situations or the resources available to cope with it (Lazarus & Folkman, 1984).

Psychological vulnerability represents potential threat. Cognitive appraisal and coping affect vulnerability and therefore individual differences that affect appraisal and coping are important determinants of psychological vulnerability (Lazarus & Folkman, 1984). Two person characteristics, namely commitments and beliefs, affect appraisal and commitments and have both cognitive and motivational components. Persons are most vulnerable in areas where they have a high commitment (cf. Lazarus & Folkman, 1984).

Beliefs influence the perception or meaning of the environments and hence influence appraisals. According to Lazarus and Folkman (1984), there are two sets of beliefs, personal control and existential. Coping may even be more essential in determining vulnerability and adaptation outcomes than appraisal. Person variables (e.g., personal resources such as health and energy) may directly affect coping.

Stress, Vulnerability, and Anxiety Research

Stress is a key concept with respect to vulnerability, anxiety, and health. Some of the earliest research on stress focused on the effects of extreme environments. Grinker and Spiegel (1945) investigated the effects of the stress of flying combat mission during World War II, on both physical and psychological functioning. Even under these severe stressful conditions, individual differences were highly relevant in determining the outcome. Grinker and Spiegel concluded that those men who became psychiatric casualities could be divided into two groups: (1) those who developed severe symptoms after exposure to minimal stress, and (2) those who developed symptoms after exposure to severe/prolonged stress. Therefore, some other factor, in addition to the stressful experiences, contributed to the occurrence of symptoms of anxiety.

Studies of natural and man-made disasters (Adams & Adams, 1984; Baum, Fleming, & Singer, 1982; Lifton & Olson, 1976) suggest that there are transient and long-term responses to stress. These would include both psychosomatic reactions and emotional reactions of anxiety, depression, anger, and feelings of helplessness. Adams and Adams (1984) studied a community located near Mount St. Helens, a volcano that erupted in May, 1980. The post-disaster stress reactions they found included increases in illness, violence, and substance abuse. The population that experienced the dam collapse and flood near Buffalo Creek, West Virginia, suffered similar effects (Lifton & Olson, 1976). The situational stress of the accident at the nuclear power plant at Three Mile Island, Pennsylvania, led to chronic, but not severe stress reactions, nor were these manifested by all respondents (Baum, Fleming, & Singer, 1982). The recent extensive nuclear accident at Chernobyl in the Soviet Union, may well have led to more severe and more widespread stress reactions.

Bonkalo (1984), after reviewing studies on transient and situational disorders in response to surgery, assault, environmental catastrophes, bereavement, or combat, has suggested that the disorders are residual effects of stressful encounters. He believed that this may affect a person's vulnerability to future stressful events. This is part of a person's transactional relationship with his or her environment and is part and parcel of an ongoing and continuous process (see Fig. 2.1).

Stressful Life Events and Illness

One area of research that has been prominent, especially in the last 10 years, has been that concerned with stressful life events (Dohrenwend & Dohrenwend, 1978, 1981; Holmes & Rahe, 1967; Rabkin & Struening, 1976). However, the general concept goes back at least to Meyer, in a paper he presented on "The Contributions of Psychiatry to the Understanding of Life Problems" on May 26, 1921 (see Lief, 1948). Some of the early research in this area was started by Hinkle and his co-workers in the 1950s (see Hinkle & Plummer, 1952; Hinkle & Wolff, 1957a, 1957b, 1958; Hinkle, 1962). They were the first to attempt large-scale studies of the relationship between life events and illness. Their work on telephone company employees is summarized by Minter and Kimball (1980). These studies covered up to 20 years, and Hinkle and his co-workers found that: ". . . (1) a small number of people (25 percent) have most of the illness episodes (50 percent). (2) As the number of illness episodes increase, the number of organ systems involved also increases (thus, chronic diseases did not bias the results). (3) As the number of episodes of illness increase, the individual exhibits an increased number of etiologies of illness. (4) As the number of episodes of illness increases, the number of disturbances in mood, thought and behavior also increases. (5) Clusters of illness, which were composed of several 'different and ostensibly unrelated syndromes,' were observed to occur and were not related to activity, diet, rest or exposure to infections. (6) Such clusters of illness occurred most often when a person had a life situation described as unsatisfactory or when he experienced difficulty in adapting to his environment" (Minter & Kimball, 1980, pp. 190–191).

Hinkle and Plummer (1952) also discovered that absences from work because of illness were due to a small number of people. The "high-absence" group, compared to the "low-absence" group, suffered from more major and minor illness, injuries, operations, as well as emotional disturbances and thinking and behavioral problems. They also had more conflicts and anxieties, were unhappy and discontented, and were difficult to supervise. Furthermore, they had been subjected to more stressful experiences and situations. In effect, Hinkel and his co-workers were pioneers in the investigation of the relationship between stressful life events and illness, although they did not quantify their assessment of life events.

The first quantitative measure of life-change events was developed by Holmes and Rahe and their colleagues. They initially developed the Schedule of Recent Experience (SRE), consisting of 43 life-change events ranging from minor law violations to death of a spouse (Holmes & Rahe, 1967). These events were found to cause a person to make some type of life adjustment. They then refined this measure according different weights to different life events and developed the Social Readjustment Rating Scale (SRRS) (Holmes & Rahe, 1967). The weights were empirically derived in terms of the amount of adjustment needed for the event (Masuda & Holmes, 1967). The amount of life change, or Life Change Unit (LCU), was determined by multiplying the weight for each event by its frequency within a given time period. Positive but low correlations between LCUs and psychological distress or illness have been reported in the literature by a number of investigator (e.g., Dohrenwend & Dohrenwend, 1978; Gunderson & Rahe, 1974); Rabkin & Struening, 1976).

The general conclusions drawn from the various studies include: (a) stressful life events preceded the onset of illness; (b) most of the illnesses (about 4 out of 5) were minor; (c) most of the illness episodes were due to a small percentage of people; (d) demographic factors played a role (e.g., high incidence in younger men, blacks, unmarried men, men with less education and high job dissatisfaction). Illness data are often based on self-reports.

A major difficulty of the early studies is that there was no assessment of the significance or meaning of a particular life event. For one woman, a divorce may be liberating; for another, it may cause undue hardship. For one man, the death of a spouse who has suffered from cancer may be a relief; for another, it may be earth shattering. Yet all these events would be weighted equally on the SRRS. Critical evaluation of the life-change event research indicates that persons may perceive and respond to the same objective event quite differently (cf. Antonovsky, 1974).

Sarason, Johnson, and Siegel (1978) developed a Life Experiences Survey to measure life changes, which eliminates some problems associated with the other life-change scales. Their scale assesses both positive and negative life experiences, and provides for individualized ratings of the impacts of events. The authors point out that it is important to assess the role of moderator variables in affecting the relationship between stressful life events and illness. Furthermore, they state 'that one's perception of control over environmental events, sensation-seeking status, and a degree of psychosocial assets may all mediate the effects of life stress" (Sarason et al. 1978).

Paykel (1983), after reviewing the methodology for life-event research, offered three conclusions. (1) With respect to data collection, he believes that self-report event questionnaires are inadequate for the 1980s; interview methods should be used. (2) "Events should be documented in relation to the time of illness onset, and in some ways those events unlikely to be caused by illness should be considered separately" (p. 350). (3) With respect to data analyses or quantification, Paykel believes that not all life events are equal, therefore, it is necessary to develop alternative methods to distinguish more stressful events from less stressful events.

Endler and Edwards (in press) indicate that two important trends have evolved in the stressful life-events literature, as a result of critical evaluations of previous research: There has recently been an assessment of (1) dimensions of appraisal and (2) individual difference variables (e.g., vulnerability) that affect the perception of a response to stressful events that have been investigated.

According to Endler and Edwards, (in press), individual differences in vulnerability can be conceptualized in at least three ways: (1) in terms of cognitive factors (e.g., Kobasa, 1979; Lefcourt, 1980); (2) in terms of response predispositions in interaction with a specific range of situations (e.g., Endler, 1975, 1980, 1983; Chesney & Rosenman, 1983; and (3) in terms of the interaction process (Lazarus & Folkman, 1984). Let us briefly discuss some of the research from each of these perspectives.

Cognitive Factors and Vulnerability to Stressors

Kobasa (1979) has indicated that the correlations between life events and illness, although positive, are not very large. She has postulated "hardiness" as a personality characteristic, differentiating individuals who do not become ill as a result of high levels of stress experience from those who do become ill due to stress. Hardy persons believe they can *control* or influence stressful events they experience and have the ability to feel deeply committed to their life activities. They perceive change as an exciting challenge that enables them to develop. They do not perceive change and life events as detrimental. Her research and that of others, studies of business executives in highly stressful work environments, support the hypothesis relating hardiness to illness (Kobasa, 1979; Kobasa, Maddi, & Kahn, 1982; Kobasa & Puccetti, 1983). Hardiness affects both appraisal of an event and coping strategies in negotiating that event. Hardiness, via cognitive appraisal, enables the person to transform a stressful experience into a less stressful form rather than avoiding the situation.

Another factor that influences vulnerability to potential stress is perceived control (a cognitive expectancy) (Rotter, 1966; Phares, 1976; Lefcourt, 1980). Glass and Singer (1972) found that perception of control in a stressful situation can minimize its negative effects.

Locus of control (Rotter, 1966, 1975) influences coping activities and emotional response to stressors (Phares, 1976). Internals both seek and use more information than externals (Davis & Phares, 1967; Seeman, 1963; Seeman & Evans, 1962). Lefcourt (1980) found that internals differ from externals on coping strategies (e.g., humor) and that externals manifest more tension than internals when faced with acheivement related failures.

Johnson and Sarason (1979) proposed that locus of control may *mediate* the effects of life change. They found a significant modest positive correlation between both anxiety and depression, and negative life change events for externals, but not for internals. According to Lefcourt, Martin, and Saleh (1984), locus of control for social interaction moderates the relationships among life events, social support, and mood.

Interaction of Temperament and Environment

Interest in the relationship between temperament and personality would appear to be growing within psychology (Strelau, Farley, & Gale, 1985). Thomas, Chess, and Birch (1970) have examined the nature of temperamental differences in children and their interaction with environmental influences in personality formation. They suggest that there are constitutional differences in temperament that, when interacting with the environment, shape personality. Observing children from birth and also interviewing their parents over a number of years, they observed the children's development up to and including the preschool period, nursery school, and elementary school. On the basis of their research, they have been able to identify three general types or clusters of temperament: "easy children," "difficult children," and "slow-to-warm-up children." They suggest that a different style of child-rearing practice is most appropriate for each of these three types. Their major point, however, is that personality development is a function of the interaction of constitutional temperament factors and environmental influences. Thomas, Chess, and Birch suggest that parent-child interactions are bidirectional, which is similar to Bell's proposition that parents' socializing practices have an effect on children, but also that children's individual characteristics (determined by congenital and environmental factors) influences the parents' behavior.

Strelau (1983) suggests that temperament dimensions (e.g., activity, mobility) may be determined directly by an individual's biological endowment. Although this endowment is inherited, particular dimensions may develop and change under environmental influences. Normally, temperament plays a minor role in influencing the general development of personality. However, extreme environmental factors (e.g., overstimulation or deprivation) may dramatically increase the role played by temperament in personality development.

Vulnerability and the Interaction Between Traits and Situations

The Endler multidimensional interaction model of anxiety (Endler, 1975, 1980, 1983) postulates that increased in state anxiety are due to the interactions between a specific facet of trait anxiety (e.g., social evaluation) and a *congruent* stressful situation (e.g, a job interview).

A series of studies by Endler and his students (Endler, 1985; Endler, Edwards, & Vitelli, 1985, in press) and by others (e.g, Kendall, 1978) empirically supports the differential hypothesis. They have found interactions for congruent trait-situation dimensions and no interactions for noncongruent trait-situations dimensions. Endler and Okada (1975), in a laboratory experiment, noted changes in state anxiety in female students as a result of an interaction between physical danger A-trait and a physical danger stressor (threat of electric shock). No interactions were found between the physical danger situations and the noncongruent dimensions of trait anxiety, such as social evaluation. Endler, Edwards, and Kowalchuk (1983) investigated the interaction model of anxiety in short-term psychotherapy situations involving both male and female patients. There was a significant interaction between the "social evaluation" psychotherapy situations and social evaluation A-trait in predicting A-state *decrease* during therapy and an interaction for the ambiguous A-trait for females. There were also interactions for both sexes for innocuous A-trait.

Endler, Edwards, and McGuire (1979) studied anxiety in male and female actors in metropolitan Toronto, both during rehearsal and prior to an important stage performance, and found a trend toward a significant interaction between social evaluation A-trait and the congruent situational stressor of a stage performance in eliciting A-state changes. Unfortunately, the sample size was small.

Endler, King, Edwards, Kuczynski, and Diveky (1983) reported a significant social evaluation A-trait by on-the-job social evaluation stress in eliciting A-trait changes for middle-management bankers.

Flood and Endler (1980) examined the interaction model of anxiety in a real-life track meet competition, and Endler, King, and Herring (1985) studied a karate competition. Both studies found interactions between social evaluation A-trait and congruent social evaluation stress in eliciting increases in A-state.

Endler and Magnusson (1977) investigated the interaction model of anxiety in a real-life classroom examination situation with Swedish college students. Phillips and Endler (1982) conducted a similar study with Canadian college students and Endler, King, Kuczynski, and Edwards (1980) replicated this study with Canadian high-school students. Endler and Magnusson (1977) found a significant interaction between interpersonal A-trait and the exam situation stress in eliciting increases in pulse rate (an index of A-state). Endler and co-workers (1980) and Phillips and Endler (1982) found significant social evaluation A-trait by exam stress interaction in evoking increases in A-state.

Type A behavior patterns are analogous to response predispositions (e.g., A-trait) that interact with stressful situations. As originally conceptualized (Friedman & Rosenman, 1974), Type A was not a personality type or trait but a set of behaviors that are derived from an *interaction* between a challenging environment and personal predispositions. According to Chesney and Rosenman (1983), the Type A behavior pattern includes "such behavioral dispositional as ambitiousness, aggressiveness, competitiveness and impatience; specific behaviors such as alertness, muscle tenseness, rapid and emphatic speech stylistics; and emotional reactions such as enhanced irritation and expressed signs of anger" (p. 548). The Type A behavior pattern involves a chronic struggle with time, with the aim being to accomplish more and more in less and less time, and by competition with other persons or environmental forces (Chesney & Rosenman, 1983). Type A behavior should be manifested in predisposed persons by situations in which their control is challenged.

The positive relationship between Type A behavior and coronary heart diseases (CHD) was first demonstrated in the Western Collaborative Study (cf. Chesney & Rosenman, 1983). Type A persons manifest greater sympathetic nervous system and cardiovascular arousal when threatened by stressors than do Type B persons (Dembroski, MacDougall, & Shields, 1977; Glass et al., 1980). Aspects of the situation, however, are important in evoking these differences in Type A versus Type B persons. Those situations that emphasize a challenge or involve harassment magnify the response differences between Type A and Type B persons (Glass et al., 1980).

The original Type A concept was a composite of a number of behaviors including ambitiousness, aggressiveness, competitiveness, and impatience. More recently, there is evidence that some components, such as hostility (Chesney & Rosenman, 1983) and cynicism (Williams, 1984), may be especially important in evoking the perception of challenge and Type A behavior. Fischman (1987) has recently summarized the Type A literature. Recent studies have not always found a relationship between Type A behavior pattern and CHD. There may be two major reasons for this. First, the paper and pencil questionnaires used for assessing Type A may not get at the nuances and subtleties that are evoked by the Structured Interview Method. Second, Type A seems to be a multidimensional concept. Williams (1984) has concluded that the basic factor relating Type A to CHD may not be Type A behavior per se but rather a cynical, mistrusting attitude. Chesney and Rosenman (1983) believe that "true risk has less to do with the 'hurry sickness' than it does with the potential for hostility . . ." (Fischman, 1987, p. 50). Check and Dyck (1986) found that Type A persons are more aggressive than Type Bs, and report a greater desire to hurt others. Chesney and Rosenman (1983) propose that it is important to investigate the interactions between characteristics of the situation and of the individual in eliciting the *perception* of challenge. Furthermore, they believe that it is neccessary to do research on the dynamic interaction process. Specifically, research should focus on the coping styles used by individuals who differ in Type A and Type B behavior patterns in challenging situations.

Another important individual difference predisposition related to stress, is sensation seeking (Zuckerman, 1974). Sensation seeking refers to a tendency to prefer, seek out, and enjoy highly varied, stimulating, and exciting situations. High sensation seekers may respond quite differently to life-change events than low sensation seekers (Johnson & Sarason, 1979). High sensation seekers seem to be less aroused and better able to cope with change. Smith, Johnson, and Sarason (1978) have found correlations between negative life changes and adjustment problems for low sensation (or arousal) seekers but not for high sensation seekers.

Vulnerability and Dynamic Process Variables

Lazarus's theory and research, and that of his colleagues, emphasize the importance of focusing on the *process* involved in stress, especially appraisal and coping strategies (Lazarus & Folkman, 1984). Lazarus and Launier (1978) have indicated the importance of the mediating role of cognitive appraisal in the stress-anxiety process. A person's level of arousal is influenced by his or her cognitive appraisal of the situations.

Folkman and Lazarus (1985) examined the coping process at three stages of a stressful examination situation in college students. They state that a stressful encounter is a dynamic unfolding process with the essence of stress, coping, and adaptation being *change*. They found significant changes in emotion and coping across the three stages and noted that individuals experienced contradictory emotions (e.g., both threat and challenge emotions) and cognitions during each stage. "Finally, despite normatively shared emotion reactions at each stage, substantial individual differences remained" (Folkman & Lazarus, 1985, p. 150). Edwards, Lay, Parker, and Endler (1987) did a similar study with grade-13 high-school students and found, in general, that the main effects of the stage variable paralleled the Folkman and Lazarus (1985) normative data. Edwards and co-workers (1987) also found that procrastination, social evaluation A-trait, and stage variables (trials) interacted, so that the high procrastination, high trait-anxious subjects were the most state axious during the preparation stages, but least anxious at Stage 3 (post- examination). State anxiety and trait anxiety were assessed via the Endler Multidimensisonal Anxiety Scales (EMAS) (Endler, Edwards, & Vitelli, in press).

The state form of the EMAS scales yields two subscale scores, representing the autonomic-emotional component of state anxiety and the cognitive-worry component of state anxiety. Both of these scores are combined to produce a total state-anxiety scale score. The EMAS trait inventory is a trait anxiety measure that assesses separately four types of general situations: one in which a person is being evaluated by other people, another that involves or may involve physical danger, a third involving a new or strange situation, and one that involves one's daily routines. The third EMAS scale assesses whether persons perceive particular situations to be a social-evaluation situation, physical-danger situation, ambiguous situation, or innocuous situation. The stress, coping, adaptation, and anxiety process is highly complex and different relationships may occur at different stages in the process. For example, in a study now in progress, we assessed college students on A-trait and A-state at three stages; two weeks before a psychology exam (Stage 1, nonstress); prior to the exam (Stage 2, stress) and a few weeks after the exam, but just before they received their exam results (Stage 3, stress). Table 2.1 presents the *p* levels of significance for some of our results on A-State.

It is obvious that the situational stressor of the anticipation of the exam and anticipation of the results of the exam was effective in producing changes in A-state. The anxiety level increased prior to the exam and decreased after the exam. A-trait (high versus low) only had an effect when comparing Stages 1 and 2. The interaction of social evaluation A-trait and situational stress was only effective on the cognitive component of A-state when comparing Stages 1 and 3, that is two weeks prior to the exam (non-stress) versus post-exam but prior to receiving the results (stress). Table 2.2 presents the means relevant to this interaction.

The high social evaluation A-trait students decreased their cognitive A-state; the low A-Trait students increased their cognitive A-state. Initially

Table 2.1. State Anxiety (A-State) During Three Stages of an Examination Process*

Sources of Variance	Stages 1, 2, 3 A-State			Stages 1 vs 2 A-State			Stages 1 vs 3 A-State			Stages 2 vs 3 A-State		
	C	E	T	C	E	T	C	E	T	C	E	T
A-Trait (social evaluation)				.033	.033	.021						
Gender (sex)				.003	.039	.005						
Situation (stage)	<.001	<.001	<.001							<.001	<.001	<.001
A-Trait × Stage†							.016					

p Levels of Significance

*p values based on an analysis of variance.
† The results for the A-Trait × Sex interaction and the Sex × Stage × A-Trait interaction were not significant.

Notes:

1. Stage 1 = Non-Stress—Two weeks before exam.
2. Stage 2 = Stress—Prior to exam.
3. Stage 3 = Stress—Post-exam, but prior to receiving results.
4. A-Trait classification is based on top 40% and bottom 40% on social evaluation A-Trait.
5. Gender = sex = males versus females.
6. A-State: C = Cognitive Worry Component.
   E = Autonomic Emotional Component.
   T = Total State Anxiety Score.

Table 2.2. Means on Cognitive A-State for College Students*

Variables	Mean Cognitive A-State Stages	
Social Evaluation A-Trait (SE)	Stage 1 (non-stress)	Stage 3 (stress)
High SE (top 40%)	15.0 (N = 43, F = 28, M = 15)	13.0 (N = 43, F = 28, M = 15)
Low SE (bottom 40%)	12.5 (N = 37, F = 22, M = 15)	13.1 (N = 37, F = 22, M = 15)

*Two weeks prior to an exam (Stage 1) and post-exam but prior to receiving exam results (Stage 3).

Table 2.3. Correlations Between Social Evaluation A-Trait and Psychology Grades for College Students*

r		Difference Z Score
Females	Males	
.35†	−.20	2.54‡

* Female (N = 49); male (N = 28).
† $p < .01$
‡ $p < .02$

(Stage 1) the high A-trait students manifested significantly more A-state than low A-trait students. After the exam, there were no cognitive A-state differences between the two groups.

We also correlated the students anxiety scores with their grades for females, social evaluation A-Trait was significantly correlated with grades $r = .35$ ($p < .01$); for males the correlation between these two variables was −.20. The difference between these two correlations was significant: $Z = 2.54$, $p < .02$. For females social evaluation A-Trait was positively correlated with grades; for males these two variables were negatively correlated (see Table 2.3).

Females achieve better grades when they are high on social evaluation A-Trait; for males the reverse seems to be true. Greenglass (1985) has suggested that "women are interpreting most situations they encounter, even their daily routines are socially evaluative" (p. 47). It may be that because they perceive every situation as socially evaluative and anxiety provoking, the anxiety is the factor that motivates them to get good grades and do well in their jobs—the factor that motivates them to achieve. For males high levels of anxiety may be debilitating in terms of achievement. Greenglass (1982), in discussing Matina Horner's (1972) research on the motivation to avoid success in women, suggests that perhaps women's expectations for success are lower than men's, and that women are expected to be less competent than men. We would suggest that if they perceive themselves as less competent they may become anxious when they do perform competently.

Hassles

Much of the research on the effects of stress on illness has focused on major stressful life events, such as divorce, marriage, retirement, death of a spouse or child, birth of a child, and losing one's job. In recent years the role of minor stressful life events or hassles has been investigated. Hassles would include such daily life experiences as waiting in line, being stuck in a traffic jam, misplacing or losing something, doing household chores, being in the presence of an inconsiderate smoker, tearing one's clothes, and having a dispute with a colleague at work. These hassles may have an impact on illness and health via their cumulative impact or they may affect the relationship between major life events and illness. For example, if a major life stressful event (e.g., divorce) occurs when minor hassles are at a minimum, the stress may not be as detrimental as when hassles are at a premium. At other times hassles may be the "straw that breaks the camel's back."

Lazarus and his colleagues (Lazarus, 1984; Kanner, Coyne, Schaefer, & Lazarus, 1981) have recently developed a daily hassles scale one that measures minor stressful life events. The scale is a mixture of different categories including *environmental events* (e.g., inconsiderate smokers), disappointing or worrisome *chronic environmental conditions* (e.g. rising prices), *ongoing worries or concern* (e.g., job dissatisfactions), and *distressed emotional reactions* (e.g., fear of rejection) (cf. Lazarus, 1984). The scale also included measures of uplifts, pleasant of satisfying daily events (e.g. eating out, getting enough sleep, completing a task).

Kanner and colleagues (1981) found the intensity and frequency of hassles were a better predictor of psychological and physical symptoms of illness and health than major life events. Cohen and Hoberman (1983) reported that positive life events (uplifts) lessened psychological distress and physical symptoms for those persons who experienced a high amount of stress. Lazarus (1981) notes that "contrary to our expectation, uplifts did not seem to have much buffer effect on the impact of hassles. . . . In fact, for women, uplifts seemed to have negative effects on emotions and on psychological health" (p. 62).

Dohrenwend and Shrout (1985) suggest that the Hassles Scale is confounded with symptoms of psychological distress, and that is why the Hassles Scale correlates so highly with the Hopkins Symptoms Check List, the index used by Lazarus and his colleagues to assess health and illness. Lazarus, De Longis, Folkman, and Gruen (1985) note that appraisal is part of stress assessment. Be that as it may, it is obvious that hassles and stressful life events can and do affect health and illness. What is needed, on the one hand, is a revision of hassle scales that focuses on the meaning or appraisal of hassles, and on the other hand, an objective index of illness, rather than a check list to assess health. Furthermore, what is needed is a fine-grained (micro) analysis of hassles and their dynamic interaction with antecedent and consequent events.

Stress, Biochemical Changes, and Illness

We have been discussing the effects of stressful life events and hassles on illness and health. What affect does stress have on a biochemical changes, and what effects do these changes have on illness and on health? As indicated earlier when a threat is perceived, there is increased action in the autonomic nervous system and endocrine systems; the body is aroused and motivated. There is an increased in heart rate, in blood pressure, respiration, and blood sugar level. Furthermore, there is a secretion of catecholamines circulation to the muscles is increased and circulation of blood to the skin is reduced.

According to Pert (1981), there is evidence that psychological stress leads to the release of endorphins. "Researchers at the Max Planck Institute in Germany, for example, have found a significant increase in the levels of endorphins in the blood of university students who are about to take important examinations" (p. 100). The brain in response to physical pain and psychological stress releases endorphins, which serve as a natural analgesic, and may induce a feeling of euphoria. Whereas increased adrenalin due to stress increases heart rate, blood pressure, and metabolism, the endorphins slow respiration, lower blood pressure, and calm motor activity. The release of endorphins due to stress, thus, has adaptive value.

Stressful experiences and life events also effect the autoimmune system. Bartrop, Lazarus, Kiloh, and Penny (1977) have investigated the effects of bereavement on surviving spouses in New South Wales, Australia, examining emotional consequences and physical health, especially the body's capability to stave off disease. Among other findings, they noted that the immune systems of bereaved spouses were weakened and they had lower activity levels of T cells (blood cells that defend against and attack foreign substances). Ornstein and Sobel (1987) report on a study conducted at the Mount Sinai School of Medicine (New York), which found that men married to women with terminal breast cancer manifested a "drop in responsiveness of the lymphocytes (another of the blood cells specialized for defense) immediately after their wives' deaths, a drop that continued for two months" (p. 50). However, the husband's immune functioning recovered between 4 and 14 months after the spouse's death; a change congruent with the change in the psychological state.

Ornstein and Sobel also suggest that the cells of the immune system respond to chemical signals (e.g., catecholamines, prostaglandins, thyroid hormones, serotonin, and endorphins) from the central nervous system.

Psychological and physical stress release neurohormones that subsequently affect the immune system. Increases in levels of circulating hormones suppress immune fuctions, and stresses and hassles seem to be associated with decreases in levels of immune cell activity. Ornstein and Sobel also report on some studies that indicate that positive and enjoyable experiences may enhance immunity and even relaxation training can improve cellular immune fuction.

Maier and Laudenslager (1985) point out that in addition to stress causing ulcers, there is now evidence that vulnerability to infectious disease, and possibly even cancer, may be influenced by how people react to stress. Not everyone exposed to or infected by identifiable pathogens (e.g., viruses and bacteria) become ill, and thus psychological factors may have an important effect in determining who does and who does not become ill.

It may be that persons who can *control* negative circumstances showed greater immunity to disease; those who cannot control their stressful situations become less immune to disease and illness. Locke, Hurst, Heisel, Kraus, and Williams (1979) found that persons who had many life stresses plus high levels of anxiety and depression had the lowest level of natural killer (NK) cells (part of the lymphocyte family) activity, and hence, a decrease in the functioning of the immune system. Persons with high life stresses, but low levels of anxiety and depression had the highest level of NK-cell activity. This suggests to Locke and colleagues that those persons who can cope with stress have high NK-cell activity and are more immune to disease than those who respond with anxiety and depression reflecting their poor coping skills and leading to lowered NK-cell activity.

Similarly, Levy (1983), in her study of women with breast cancer, found that the women who passively accepted the disease manifested lower NK-cell activity than those women who responded with anger and agitation. Passive acceptance is a helpless reaction and lowers the level of functioning of the immune system. Anger and agitation involve attempts at control, increase the level of functioning of the immune system, and slow down the course of the disease. Obviously, psychological factors can, and do affect physical illness (see Fig. 2.1).

Happiness and Optimism

As indicated above, control seems to mitigate the behavioral effects of stress and also minimizes the probability of physical illness and disease.

Thompson (1981), in a review of the literature on the control over a stressful event and the degree of ensuing psychological stress or pain, notes that when persons believe they can control the administration of a stressor, they will find the stressor less unpleasant than people who do not believe they have this control. She points out that "reactions to potentially stressful events depend on their meaning for the individual"(p. 89). Goodhart (1985) found that "negative thinking about prior stressor outcomes appeared to increase vulnerability to the impact of later ones on several aspects of well-being" (p. 216). Positive thinking, however, appears to have minimal long-term effect. "Rather, it appears that the absence of negative thinking, not the presence of positive thinking, could be more beneficial" (pp. 230–231). Perhaps, Pollyanna and Norman Vincent Peale were only partially correct.

Jones (1986) suggests that expectancies influence both how we perceive reality and the reality itself. Scheier, Weintraub, and Carver (1986) found that optimists cope with stress better than pessimists. They found that optimists react to disappointments (e.g., not getting into graduate school) by consulting with other people and developing a plan of action in order to cope with the problem. Pessimists, on the other hand, react by "giving up" or trying to forget about their rejections. Seligman (see Trotter, 1987) believes that the manner in which individuals usually explain their failures to themselves affects both their achievements and their health. Pessimists perceive failures (e.g., failing an exam) as being due to personal deficiencies and are also more susceptable to disease, illness, and infection than optimists (cf. Peterson & Seligman, 1984). According to Trotter (1987), Seligman believes that explanatory style ". . . can change in response to important events in one's life, including psychotherapy. And he believes that cognitive therapy is the best approach, since it assumes that depression is a result of distorted thinking about the world (global), the future (stable) and oneself (internal)" (p. 39).

Bandura (1986) on the basis of his research, concludes that *self-efficacy* (a belief in one's ability to cope with specific situations) affects a person's stress reactions and his or her consequent behavior. Persons high on self-efficacy can better cope with stress and can lead healthier lives. Presumably, they will also be happier people.

Conclusions

The relationships among anxiety, stress, and coping and their relationship to health, illness, and happiness are highly complex. There is a dynamic interaction among all these factors (see Figure 2.1) and how a person perceives a stressful situation is an important determinant of how he or she will cope with it. Individuals who perceive themselves as being able to control stressful situations and who have a high sense of self-efficacy in terms of being able to learn to master life's problems should be able to minimize their levels of stress and anxiety, and should be able to maximize their coping skills. These individuals should be happier and healthier persons.

Acknowledgments. Preparation of this chapter was supported in part by Social Sciences and Humanities Research Council of Canada Grant 410-84-1261 to the author.

The author gratefully acknowledges the assistance of James Parker for his comments and suggestions about the manuscript, for compiling the references, and for some of the data analyses. Thanks are due also to Romeo Vitelli for statistical analyses, to Janet Clewes, Brian Cox, and Dean Crooks for assistance in collecting some of the data. Professor Doug McCann made his Introductory Psychology students available to participate in the classroom examination study described in the chapter.

References

Adams, P.R., & Adams, G.R. (1984). Mount Saint Helen's ashfall: Evidence for a disaster stress reaction. *American Psychologist, 39*, 252–260.

Alexander, F.G., & Selesnick, S.T. (1966). *The History of Psychiatry*. New York: Harper & Row.

American Psychiatric Association. (1980). *Diagnostic and statistical manual of mental disorders* (3rd ed.). Washington, DC: Author.

Antonovsky, A. (1974). Conceptual and methodological problems in the study of resistance resources and stressful life events. In B.S. Dohrenwend & B.P. Dohrenwend (Eds.), *Stressful life events: Their nature and effects* (pp. 245–258). Toronto: John Wiley & Sons.

Appley, M.H., & Trumbull, R. (1967). *Psychological stress: Issues in research*. New York: Appleton-Century-Crofts.

Bandura, A. (1982). Self-efficacy mechanism in human agency. *American Psychologist, 37*, 122–147.

Bandura, A. (1986). *Social foundations of thought and action: A social cognitive theory*. Englewood Cliffs, NJ: Prentice Hall.

Bartrop, R.W., Lazarus, L., Kiloh, L.G., & Penny, R., (1977). Depressed lymphocyte function after bereavement. *Lancet, 1*, No. 8016, 834–836.

Baum, A., Fleming, R., & Singer, J.E. (1982). Stress at Three Mile Island: Applying psychological impact analysis. In L. Bickman (Ed.), *Applied social psychology annual* (Vol. 3, pp. 217–248). Beverly Hills, CA: Sage.

Bonkalo, A. (1984). Transient and situational disorders. In N.S. Endler & J. McV. Hunt (Eds.), *Personality and the behavioral disorders* (Vol. 2, 2nd ed., pp. 897–913). New York: John Wiley & Sons.

Cannon, W.B. (1932). *The wisdom of the body*. New York: Norton.

Cattell, R.B., & Scheier, I.H. (1961). *The meaning and measurement of neuroticism and anxiety*. New York: The Ronald Press.

Check, J.V.P., & Dyck, D.G. (1986). Hostile aggression and Type A behavior. *Personality and Individual Differences, 7*, 819–827.

Chesney, M.A., & Rosenman, R.H. (1983). Specificity in stress models: Examples drawn from Type A Behavior. In C.L. Cooper (Ed.), *Stress research: Issues for the eighties* (pp. 21–34). Toronto: John Wiley & Sons.

Chess, S., Thomas, A., & Birch, H.G. (1976). Behavior problems revisited: Findings of an anterospective study. In N.S. Endler, L.R. Boulter, & H. Osser (Eds.), *Contemporary issues in developmental psychology* (2nd ed., pp. 562–568). Toronto: Holt, Rinehart & Winston.

Cohen, S., & Hoberman, H.M. (1983). Positive events and social supports as buffers of life change stress. *Journal of Applied Social Psychology, 13*, 99–125.

Coyne, J.C., & Lazarus, R.S. (1980). Cognitive style, stress perception and coping. In I.L. Kutash & L.B. Schlesinger (Eds.), *Handbook on stress and anxiety: Contemporary knowledge, theory and treatment* (pp. 144–158). San Francisco: Jossey-Bass Publishers.

Davis, W.L., & Phares, E.J. (1967). Internal-external control as a determinant of information-seeking in a social influence situation. *Journal of Personality, 35,* 547–561.

Dembroski, T.M., MacDougall, J.M., & Shields, T.L. (1977). Physiological reactions to social challenge in persons evidencing Type A coronary-prone behavior pattern. *Journal of Human Stress, 3,* 2–10.

Dohrenwend, B.S., & Dohrenwend, B.P. (1978). Some issues in research on stressful life events. *The Journal of Nervous and Mental Disease, 166,* 7–15.

Dohrenwend, B.S., & Dohrenwend, B.P. (1981). Life stress and illness: Formulations of the issues. In B.S. Dohrenwend & B.P. Dohrenwend (Eds.), *Stressful life events and their contexts* (pp. 1–27). New York: Prodist.

Dohrenwend, B.P., & Shrout, P.E. (1985). "Hassles" in the conceptualization and measurement of life stress variables. *American Psychologist 40,* 780–785.

Dollard, J., & Miller, N.E. (1950). *Personality and psychotherapy: An analysis in terms of learning, thinking and culture.* New York: McGraw-Hill.

Edwards, J.M., & Endler N.S. (1983). Personality research. In M. Hersen, A.E. Kazdin, & A.S. Bellack (Eds.), *The clinical psychology handbook* (pp. 223–238). New York: Pergamon Press.

Edwards, J.M., Lay, C.H., Parker, S.D., & Endler, N.S. (1987). The relationship of procrastination and trait-anxiety to measures of emotion and coping during three stages of an examination period. Department of Psychology Reports, York University, Toronto, No. 163.

Endler, N.S. (1975). A person-situation interaction model of anxiety. In C.D. Spielberger & I.G. Sarason (Eds.), *Stress and anxiety* (Vol. 1., pp. 145–164). Washington, DC: Hemisphere Publishing Corporation (Wiley).

Endler, N.S. (1978). The interaction model of anxiety: Some possible implications. In D.M. Landers & R.W. Christina (Eds.), *Psychology of motor behavior and sport—1977* (pp. 332–351). Champaign, IL: Human Kinetics.

Endler, N.S. (1980). Person-situation interaction and anxiety. In I.L. Kutash & L.B. Schlesinger (Eds.), *Handbook on stress and anxiety: Contemporary knowledge, theory and treatment* (pp. 249–266). San Francisco: Jossey-Bass Publishers.

Endler, N.S. (1982). *Holiday of Darkness.* New York: John Wiley & Sons (xv + 169 pp.)

Endler, N.S. (1983). Interactionism: A personality model, but not yet a theory. In M.M. Page (Ed.), *Nebraska Symposium on Motivation 1982: Personality—Current theory and research* (pp. 155–200). Lincoln, NE: University of Nebraska Press.

Endler, N.S. (1985). The consistency of inconsistency. In E.E. Roskam (Ed.), *Measurement and personality assessment* (pp. 339–346). Amsterdam: Elsevier Science Publishers B.V. (North Holland).

Endler, N.S., & Edwards, J. (1978). Person by treatment interactions in personality research. In L.A. Pervin & M. Lewis (Eds.), *Perspectives in interactional psychology* (pp. 141–169). New York: Plenum Press.

Endler, N.S., & Edwards, J.M. (in press). Stress and vulnerability related to anxiety disorders. In C.G. Last & M. Hersen (Eds.), *Handbook of anxiety disorders.* New York: Pergamon Press.

Endler, N.S., Edwards, J.M, & Kowalchuk, B.P. (1983). The interaction model of anxiety assessed in a psychotherapy situation. *The Southern Psychologist, l,* 168–172.

Endler, N.S., Edwards, J.M., & McGuire, A. (1979). The interaction model of anxiety: An empirical test in a theatrical performance situation. Unpublished manuscript, York University, Toronto.

Endler, N.S., Edwards, J.M., & Vitelli, R. (1985). Situation-Response General Trait Anxiety Inventory (S-R GTA) and Present Affect Reactions Questionnaire (PARQ): A manual for trait and state anxiety, *Department of Psychology Reports*, York University, Toronto, No. 152.

Endler, N.S., Edwards, J.M., & Vitelli, R. (in press). *Endler Multidimensional Anxiety Scales*. Los Angeles: Western Psychological Services.

Endler, N.S., Hunt, J.McV., & Rosenstein, A.J. (1962). An S-R Inventory of anxiousness. *Psychological Monographs, 16* (17, Whole No. 536).

Endler, N.S., King, P.R., Edwards, J.M., Kuczynski, M., & Diveky, S. (1983). Generality of the interaction model of anxiety with respect to two social evaluation field studies. *Canadian Journal of Behavioural Science, 15*, 60–69.

Endler, N.S., King, P.R., & Herring, C. (1985). Interactional anxiety and karate competition. *The Southern Psychologist, 2*, 59–62.

Endler, N.S., King, P.R., Kuczynski, M., & Edwards, J.M. (1980). Examination induced anxiety: An empirical test of the interaction model. *Department of Psychology Reports*, York University, Toronto, No. 97.

Endler, N.S., & Magnusson, D. (1976a). Multidimensional aspects of state and trait anxiety: A cross-cultural study of Canadian and Swedish college students. In C.D. Spielberger & R. Diaz-Guerrero (Eds.), *Cross-cultural anxiety* (pp. 143–172). Washington, DC: Hemisphere Publishing Corporation (Wiley).

Endler, N.S., & Magnusson D. (1976b). Personality and person by situation interactions. In N.S. Endler & D. Magnusson (Eds.), *Interactional psychology and personality* (pp. 1–25). Washington, DC: Hemisphere Publishing Corporation (Wiley).

Endler, N.S., & Magnusson D. (1976c). Toward an interactional psychology of personality, *Psychological Bulletin, 83*, 956–974.

Endler, N.S., & Magnusson, D. (1977). The interaction model of anxiety: An empirical test in an examination situation. *Canadian Journal of Behavioural Science, 9*, 101–107.

Endler, N.S., & Okada, M. (1975). A multidimensional measure of trait anxiety: The S-R inventory of general trait anxiousness. *Journal of Consulting and Clinical Psychology, 43*, 319–329.

Fischman, J. (1987). Type A on trial. *Psychology Today, 21*, 42–50.

Flood, M., & Endler, N.S. (1980). The interaction model of anxiety: An empirical test in an athletic competition situation. *Journal of Research in Personality, 14*, 329–339.

Folkman, S., & Lazarus, R.S. (1985). If it changes it must be a process: A study of emotion and coping during three stages of a college examination. *Journal of Personality and Social Psychology, 48*, 150–170.

Freud, S. (1920). *A general introduction to psychoanalysis*. New York: Boni & Liveright.

Freud, S. (1933). *New introductory lectures on psychoanalysis*. New York: Norton.

Friedman, M., & Rosenman, R.H. (1974). *Type A behavior and your heart*. New York: Knopf.

Garmezy, N. (1981). Children under stress: Perspectives on antecedents and correlates of vulnerability and resistance to psychopathology. In A.I. Rabin, L. Aronoff, A.M. Barclay, & R.A. Zucker (Eds.), *Further explorations in personality* (pp. 196–269). New York: John Wiley & Sons.

Glass, D.C., Krakoff, L.R., Contrada, R., Hilton, W.F., Kehoe, K., Mannucci, E., Collins, C., Snow, B., & Eltina, E. (1980). Effect of harassment and competition upon cardiovascular and catecholaminic responses in Type A and Type B individuals. *Psychophysiology, 17,* 453–463.

Glass, D.C., & Singer, J.E. (1972). *Urban stress: Explorations on noise and social stressors.* New York: Academic Press.

Goodhart, D.E. (1985). Some psychological effects associated with positive and negative thinking about stressful event outcomes: Was Pollyanna right? *Journal of Personality and Social Psychology, 48,* 216–232.

Greenglass, E.R. (1982). *A world of difference: Gender roles in perspective.* Toronto: John Wiley & Sons.

Greenglass, E.R. (1985). An interactional perspective on job-related stress in managerial women. *The Southern Psychologist, 2,* 42–48.

Grinker, R.R., & Spiegel, J.P. (1945). *Men under stress.* New York: McGraw-Hill.

Gunderson, E.K. & Rahe, R.H. (Eds.). (1974). *Life stress and illness.* Springfield, IL: Thomas.

Harris, W.H., & Levey, J.S. (Eds.). (1975). *The new Columbia encyclopedia* (4th ed.). New York: Columbia University Press.

Hinkle, L.E. (1962). Ecological observations of the relation of physical illness, mental illness and the social environment. *Psychosomatic Medicine, 23,* 289–296.

Hinkle, L.E., & Plummer, N. (1952). Life stress and industrial absenteeism: The concentration of illness and absenteeism in one segment of a working population. *Industrial Medicine and Surgery, 21,* 363–375.

Hinkle, L.E., & Wolff, H.G. (1957a). Health and social environment: Experimental investigations. In A. Leighton, J.A. Clausen, & R.N. Wilson (Eds.), *Exploration in Social Psychiatry* (pp. 105–135). New York: Basic Books.

Hinkle, L.E., & Wolff, H.G. (1957b). The nature of man's adaptation to his total environment and the relation of this to illness. *Archives of Internal Medicine, 99,* 442–460.

Hinkle, L.E., & Wolff, H.G. (1958). Ecological investigations of the relationship between illness, life experiences, and the social environment. *Annals of Internal Medicine, 49,* 1373–1388.

Holmes, T.H., & Rahe, R.H. (1967). The Social Readjustment Rating Scale. *Journal of Psychosomatic Research, ll,* 213–218.

Horner, M.G. (1972). Toward an understanding of achievement-related conflicts in women. *Journal of Social Issues, 28,* 157–175.

Johnson, J.H., & Sarason, I.G. (1979). Moderator variables in life stress research. In I.G. Sarason & C.D. Spielberger (Eds.), *Stress and anxiety* (Vol. 6, pp. 151–167). Washington, DC: Hemisphere Publishing Corporation (Wiley).

Jones, E.E. (1986). Interpreting interpersonal behavior: The effects of expectancies. *Science, 234,* 41–46.

Kanner, A.D., Coyne, J.C., Schaefer, C., & Lazarus, R.S. (1981). Comparison of two modes of stress measurement. Daily hassles and uplifts versus major life events. *Journal of Behavioural Medicine, 4,* 1–39.

Kendall, P.C. (1978). Anxiety: States, trait-situations? *Journal of Consulting and Clinical Psychology, 46,* 280–287.

Kobasa, S.C. (1979). Stressful life events, personality, and health: An inquiry into hardiness. *Journal of Personality and Social Psychology, 37,* 1–11.

Kobasa, S.C., Maddi, S.R., & Kahn, S. (1982). Hardiness and health: A prospective study. *Journal of Personality and Social Psychology, 42,* 168–177.

Kobasa, S.C., & Puccetti, M.C. (1983). Personality and social resources in stress resistance. *Journal of Personality and Social Psychology, 45,* 839–850.

Lazarus, R.S. (1966). *Psychological stress and the coping process.* New York: McGraw-Hill.

Lazarus, R.S. (1976). *Patterns of adjustment* (3rd ed.). New York: McGraw-Hill.

Lazarus, R.S. (1981). Little hassles can be hazardous to health. *Psychology Today, 15,* 58–62.

Lazarus, R.S. (1984). Puzzles in the study of daily hassles. *Journal of Behavioral Medicine, 7,* 375–389.

Lazarus, R.S., De Longis, A., Folkman, S., & Gruen, R. (1985). Stress and adaptation outcomes. *American Psychologist, 40,* 770–779.

Lazarus, R.S., & Folkman, S. (1984). *Stress, appraisal and coping.* New York: Springer Publishing Company.

Lazarus, R.S., & Launier, R. (1978). Stress related transactions between person and environment. In L.A. Pervin & M. Lewis (Eds.), *Perspectives in interactional psychology* (pp. 287–327). New York: Plenum Publishing Corporation.

Lefcourt, H.M. (1980). Locus of control and coping with life's events. In E. Staub (Ed.), *Personality: Basic aspects and current research* (pp. 200–235). Englewood Cliffs, NJ: Prentice Hall.

Lefcourt, H.M., Martin, R.A., & Saleh, W.E. (1984). Locus of control and social support: Interactive moderators of stress. *Journal of Personality and Social Psychology, 47,* 378–389.

Levy, S.M. (1983). Host differences in neoplastic risk: Behavioral and social contributors to disease. *Health Psychology, 2,* 21–44.

Lewis, A. (1970). The ambiguous word "anxiety." *International Journal of Psychiatry, 9,* 62–79.

Lief, A. (Ed.). (1948). *The commonsense psychiatry of Dr. Adolph Meyer.* New York: McGraw-Hill.

Lifton, R.L., & Olson, E.K. (1976). The human meaning of total disaster: The Buffalo Creek experience. *Psychiatry, 39,* 1–17.

Locke, S.E., Hurst, M.W., Heisel, S.J., Kraus, L., & Williams, M. (1979, March). The influence of stress and other psychosocial factors on human immunity. Paper presented at the American Psychosomatic Society Annual meetings, Dallas.

Mahl, G.F. (1952). Relationship between acute and chronic fear and the gastric acidity and blood sugar levels in Macca mulatta monkeys. *Psychosomatic Medicine, 14,* 182–210.

Maier, S.F., & Laudenslager, M. (1985). Stress and health: Exploring links. *Psychology Today, 19,* 44–49.

Masuda, M., & Holmes, T.H. (1967). Magnitude estimations of social readjustments. *Journal of Psychosomatic Research, ll,* 219–225.

May, R. (1950). *The meaning of anxiety.* New York: Ronald Press.

May, R. (1969). *Love and will.* New York: Norton.

Meichenbaum, D. (1983). *Coping with stress.* Toronto: John Wiley & Sons.

Millon, L. (1984). The DSM III: Some historical and substantive reflections. In N.S. Endler & J. McV. Hunt (Eds.), *Personality and the behavioral disorders* (Vol. 2, 2nd ed., pp. 675–710). Toronto: John Wiley & Sons.

Minter, R.E., & Kimball, C.P. (1980). Life events, personality traits, and illness. In I.L. Kutash & L.B. Schlesinger (Eds.), *Handbook on stress and anxiety* (pp. 189–206). San Francisco: Jossey-Bass Publishers.

Olweus, D. (1977). A critical analysis of the "modern" interactionist position. In D. Magnusson & N.S. Endler (Eds.), *Personality at the crossroads: Current issues in interaction psychology* (pp. 221–233). Hillsdale, NJ: Lawrence Erlbaum Associates.

Ornstein, R., & Sobel, D. (1987). The healing brain. *Psychology Today, 21,* 48–52.

Overton, W.F., & Reese, H.W. (1973). Models of development: Methodological implications. In J.R. Nesselroade & H.W. Reese (Eds.). *Life span developmental psychology: Methodological issues* (pp. 65–86). New York: Academic Press.

Paykel, E.S. (1983). Methodological aspects of life events research. *Journal of Psychosomatic Research, 27,* 341–352.

Pert, A. (1981). The body's own tranquilizers. *Psychology Today, 15,* 100.

Peterson, C., & Seligman, M.E.P. (1984). Causal explanations as a risk factor for depression: Theory and evidence. *Psychological Review, 91,* 347–374.

Phares, E.J. (1976). *Locus of control in personality.* Morristown, NJ: General Learning Press.

Phillips, J.B., & Endler, N.S. (1982). Academic examination and anxiety: The interaction model empirically tested. *Journal of Research in Personality, 16,* 303–318.

Rabkin, J.G., & Struening E.L. (1976). Life events, stress and illness. *Science, 194,* 1013–1020.

Rotter, J.B. (1966). Generalized expectancies for internal versus external control of reinforcement. *Psychological Monographs, 80,* (1, Whole No. 609).

Rotter, J.B. (1975). Some problems and misconceptions related to the construct of internal versus external control of reinforcement. *Journal of Consulting and Clinical Psychology, 43,* 56–67.

Sarason, I.G., Johnson, J.H., & Siegel, J.M. (1978). Assessing the impact of life changes: Development of the Life Experience Survey. *Journal of Consulting and Clinical Psychology, 46,* 932–946.

Scheier, M.F., Weintraub, J.K., & Carver, C.S. (1986). Coping with stress: Divergent strategies of optimists and pessimists. *Journal of Personality and Social Psychology, 51,* 1257–1264.

Seeman, M. (1963). Alienation and social learning in a reformatory. *American Journal of Sociology, 69,* 270–284.

Seeman, M., & Evans, J.W. (1962). Alienation and learning in a hospital setting. *American Sociological Review, 27,* 772–783.

Selye, H. (1956). *The stress of life.* New York: McGraw-Hill.

Selye, H. (1976). *The stress of life* (rev. ed.). New York: McGraw-Hill.

Singer, J.L. (1984). *The human personality.* Toronto: Harcourt, Brace, Jovanovich.

Smith, R.E., Johnson, J.H., & Sarason, I.G. (1978). Life change, the sensation seeking motivation and psychological distress. *Journal of Consulting and Clinical Psychology, 46,* 348–349.

Spielberger, C.D. (1972). Anxiety as an emotional state. In C.D. Spielberger (Ed.), *Anxiety: Current trends in theory and research* (Vol. 1, pp. 24–49). New York: Academic Press.

Spielberger, C.D. (1975). Anxiety: State-trait process. In C.D. Spielberger & I.G. Sarason, (Eds.), *Stress and anxiety* (Vol. 1, pp. 115–143). Toronto: John Wiley & Sons.

Spielberger, C.D. (1976). The nature and measurement of anxiety. In C.D. Spielberger & R. Diaz-Guerrero (Eds.), *Cross cultural anxiety* (pp. 3–12). Washington, DC: Hemisphere Publishing Corporation (Wiley).

Strelau, J. (1983). *Temperament personality activity.* New York: Academic Press.

Strelau, J., Farley, F.H., & Gale, A. (1985). *The biological bases of personality and behavior: Theories, measurement techniques, and development.* New York: Hemisphere Publishing Corp.

Sturgis, E.L. (1984). Anxiety disorders. In N.S. Endler & J. McV. Hunt (Eds.), *Personality and the behavioral disorders* (Vol. 2, 2nd ed., pp. 747–770). Toronto: John Wiley & Sons.

Taylor, S.G. (1986). *Health psychology.* New York: Random House.

Thomas, A., Chess, S., & Birch, H.G. (1970). The origin of personality. *Scientific American, 223,* 102–109.

Thompson, S.C. (1981). Will it hurt less if I can control it? A complex answer to a simple question. *Psychological Bulletin, 90,* 89–101.

Trotter, R.J. (1987). Stop blaming yourself. *Psychology Today, 21,* No. 2., 30–39.

Williams, R.B. (1984). An untrusting heart. *The Sciences, 24,* 31–36.

Wolf, S., & Wolff, H.G (1947). *Human gastric function: An experimental study of a man and his stomach.* New York: Oxford University Press.

Zuckerman, M. (1974). The sensation seeking motive. In B. Mahel (Ed.), *Progress in experimental personality research* (Vol 7., pp. 80–148). New York: Academic Press.

3

The Type A Behavior Pattern and Coronary Heart Disease: Physiological and Psychological Dimensions

Michel Pierre Janisse and Dennis G. Dyck

Janisse and Dyck concern themselves in this chapter with the Type A behavior pattern and review some central issues for the theory of Type A. They focus upon both physiological and psychological attempts to understand the behavior pattern and review three notions in particular. They begin with the concept of enhanced or exaggerated physiological responsivity on the part of Type As relative to Type Bs. This proposal holds that habitual cardiovascular overreaction during a lifetime is somehow linked to coronary heart disease. The second notion explored, continuing a theme of Endler's, is that of control. It is said that for Type As, control of their environment and the people in it is of paramount importance, and that great amounts of energy are spent by them to maintain control, or to regain it when lost. It is argued that this may explain the hypervigilance and high activity temperament of the Type A. Finally, the role of hostility in the Type A character is related to the concept of coronary-prone behavior and the need to control. Hostility has long been tied to cardiovascular disease, as shown by Rosenman in Chapter 1, but it has begun to be suspected that this is the key component of the Type A behavior pattern that makes it a *coronary-prone* pattern. With regard to control, issues about its nature are discussed, giving particular concern to how its maintenance and loss may be related to the emergence and expression of hostility in the Type A. The chapter concludes by advancing several questions about control, hostility, and the Type A behavior pattern that look to future research for answers.

—EDITOR

It has been suggested that the risk of coronary heart disease (CHD) is related to a behavior pattern known as Type A (Friedman & Rosenman, 1974). This purported relationship has generated considerable interest in recent years among both medical and psychological researchers and epidemiological evidence has been presented in a number of prospective and retrospective studies (e.g., Jenkins, Zyzanski, & Rosenman, 1971; Friedman & Rosenman, 1974; Rosenman et al., 1975). Specifically, these studies have demonstrated that the Type A pattern is associated with twice the occurrence of CHD, relative to a noncoronary-prone pattern called Type B. Furthermore, such differences are unchanged when more traditional risk factors (e.g., serum cholesterol level, systolic blood pressure, smoking, etc.) are statistically controlled, indicating the independent contribution of Type A to coronary risk.

Broadly conceived, the Type A behavior pattern refers to an action-emotion complex elicited in vulnerable individuals by environmental stressors. Three behavioral components that are said to comprise the Type A pattern are: (a) an exaggerated sense of time urgency, (b) excessive competitiveness and achievement striving, and (c) hostility and aggressiveness (Friedman, 1969). The Type B individual is said to be characterized by a relative absence of these characteristics.

The most visible difference in A/B coping styles is on an active-passive continuum. Type A behavior is an *active* coping strategy. Consistent with this view is evidence linking the behavior pattern to basal activity level as measured by standard temperament scales (Rosenman, Rahe, Borhani, & Feinleib, 1976). Other results indicate that Type As are not only more physically active than are Type Bs but they also report less fatigue after exertion (Carver, Coleman, & Glass, 1976).

Beyond the activity differences between Type As and Bs, researchers have attempted to document the more qualitative components of the behavior pattern. Specifically, a number of investigations (e.g., Dembroski, Weiss, Shields, Haynes, & Feinleib, 1978; Glass, 1977; Pittner & Houston, 1980) have sought to provide evidence for the achievement striving and time urgency components of Type A, and more recently the hostility and aggression component (Carver & Glass, 1978; Check & Dyck, 1986; Janisse, Edguer, & Dyck, 1986; Strube, Turner, Cerro, Stevens, & Hinchey, 1984). These construct validation studies have generally provided support for the time urgent and achievement dimensions of Type A but the evidence is less consistent with the hostility component; moreover, there is considerable variation among individuals classified as Type A. That is, different individuals earn their Type A classification through the manifestation of different components of the behavior pattern. Since a reanalysis of data from the Western Collaborative Group Study (Rosenman et al., 1964; Rosenman et al., 1975) by Matthews and her colleagues (see Matthews, Glass, Rosenman, & Bortner, 1977) identified the hostility dimension as the toxic component of the behavior pattern, the validation of this component is of particular importance to the hypothesized relationship between Type A and CHD.

A related yet distinctively different approach to understanding the relationship between Type A behavior and CHD has been to study physiological reaction differences among Type As and Bs. Thus, rather than focusing on the psychological or behavioral dimensions of Type A behaviors, some researchers have searched for distinctive pathophysiological responses as a potentially more fruitful strategy for identifying risk factors in CHD (e.g., Goldband, 1980). In this chapter we will selectively summarize the evidence concerning the physiological and psychological aspects of the Type A behavior pattern. By so doing, the reasonableness of various hypotheses concerning the reported relationship between Type A behavior and CHD can be reconsidered.

Physiological Dimensions of the Type A Behavior Pattern

The simple assumption that has guided much research is that Type A individuals are characterized by more reactive sympathetic nervous systems than are Type Bs. A corollary of this position is that both the behavioral features of Type A as well as certain pathophysiological manifestations (i.e., increased catecholamine and lipid levels) reflect a hyperreactive autonomic nervous system. In support of this view, it has been reported that Type A (Carruthers, 1969; Hames, Lightman, & McDonough, 1965) and angina subjects (Nestle, Verghese, & Lovell, 1967) have been found to demonstrate heightened sympathetic reactivity relative to control subjects. Moreover, the enhanced sympathetic functioning of Type As is more pronounced following exposure to such ego threats as competition, evaluation, and challenge, than to physical stressors or under resting conditions (Dembroski, MacDougall, Shields, Petillo, & Lushene, 1978; Friedman, Byers, Diamont, & Rosenman, 1975). This stimulus-specific response has most often been interpreted within the framework of a "control" hypothesis which assumes that a certain class of stimuli (ego threat stressors) elicit from Type As exaggerated attempts to control their environment (Glass, 1977; Goldband, 1980). However, most of the results are equally interpretable from other frameworks, such as Strube's (1987) recent competency appraisal hypothesis.

In a study of Type As and Bs with and without CHD, Corse, Manuck, Cantwell, Giordani, and Matthews (1982) monitored heart rate (HR), systolic blood pressure (SBP), and diastolic blood pressure (DBP) while the subjects were performing a number of difficult mental tasks. They categorized subjects as Type A or B on the basis of both the Structured Interview (SI) and the Jenkins Activity Survey (JAS) measures. They found greater SBP and DBP increases during the tasks for SI-defined Type As, but not for JAS-defined Type As.

It is clear that several physiological responses that may be involved in CHD are exaggerated in Type As. In challenging situations it has been found, for example, that Type As show greater secretion of norepinephrine (Friedman, 1969) and both blood and urinary catecholamines (Friedman et al., 1975), the latter probably predisposing the arteries to infiltration by cholesterol and other lipids. These mechanisms have been viewed by researchers (e.g., Matthews, 1982) as the physiological consequence of the need of Type As to maintain control; specifically, coping to maintain control over stressors causes increased sympathetic nervous system (SNS) activity, inducing the discharge of catecholamines (Weiss, Stone, & Harrell, 1970). This in turn causes increases in blood pressure and accelerates the rate of arterial damage, inducing myocardial lesions and facilitating the occurrence of fatal cardiac arrythmias. At the present time this assumed causal chain rests on incomplete evidence, and the role of Type A behavior in promoting CHD risk, although plausible, is even more hypothetical.

In a critical review of the literature, Houston (1983) has spoken to the evidence regarding the connection between Type A and increased physiological reactivity. His reading of the evidence suggests that Type As react with greater physiological arousal than do Type Bs, especially in settings containing incentives to *accomplish something*, and a moderate probability of failure. These effects are seen both when Type As perform alone or when they are performing in interpersonal situations. It is also generally the case that Type As are more responsive than are Type Bs in situations in which they are annoyed or harassed. Houston makes three assumptions in his interpretation of these findings. The first is that Type As may have a greater need to gain and maintain control over their environment, hence they are more aroused by threats to that control than are Type Bs. The second assumption, following from the first, is that tasks containing an incentive or a moderate probability of failure may activate the Type A's need for control. The third assumption is that the Type A's need for control stems from early learning experiences that have emphasized the importance of work achievement and fear of failure.

In our laboratory we tested two hypotheses relevant to the first of these assumptions. That is, we asked whether Type As and Bs would differentially respond to a relevant stressor (ego threat) but not to an irrelevant one (cold pressor), and whether the increased arousal of the Type As would be restricted to cardiovascular responses only, or would generalize to other autonomic nervous system measures such as pupillary responses (Malcolm, Janisse, & Dyck, 1984). Measures of heart rate and pupil size were taken during baseline and during exposure to each of two sequentially presented, but counterbalanced stress conditions: ego threat and cold pressor. The physiological measures of arousal were supplemented with repeated administrations of a self-report anxiety measure.

Three distinct findings emerged. First, JAS-defined Type A subjects had higher levels of heart rate in response to ego threat, but lower levels in response to the cold pressor, compared to their nonstressed baseline levels. On the other hand, Type B subjects had slight, but not differential heart rate increases to the two different stressful regimens. This evidence is consistent with the hypothesis that Type As respond differently to competence threatening stressors involving ego threat than they do to a physical stressor per se.

Type Bs, on the other hand, do not differentiate between ego and non-ego threatening stressors. A second finding was that the pupillary response to light did not produce results comparable to those obtained with heart rate, or with the hypothesis that Type As overall are more generally physiologically responsive than are Type Bs. Thus, it is likely that the Type A's autonomic hyperresponsiveness is not only limited to ego threatening stressors, but may also be confined to the cardiovascular portion of the autonomic nervous system. Finally, the Type A subjects in all conditions reported less anxiety than did Type B subjects. Thus, in addition to fatigue (Glass, 1977), it would appear that Type As also suppress the performance threatening subjective state of anxiety.

In general then, our results supported the notion that Type As respond differentially to ego threatening stimuli and not "stressors" in general. Further, the confinement of these A/B differences to the heart rate measure are noteworthy and indicate that a general version of the sympathetic overreaction hypothesis may be incorrect. In a similar but more general vein, it has been argued that the physiological arousal/Type A relationship is inconsistently found and is of a smaller magnitude than is generally assumed (Holmes, 1983). Following a review of the literature covered by Houston, Holmes presents a more modest conclusion, stating that only SBP has been consistently able to distinguish between Type As and Type Bs, and even here the median difference (6mm Hg) is so small as to be negligible. On the basis of his review, Holmes presents a *weak link* hypothesis. This hypothesis argues that because the relationship between Type A and CHD is, in theory, mediated by the relationship between Type A and physiological arousal, and because the relationship between Type A and physiological arousal is a weak one, the link between the Type A behavior pattern and CHD remains as unproven hypothesis. Although we fully concur with Holmes' cautionary posture, his argument confuses empirical and theoretical issues. The relationship between Type A behavior and CHD is an empirical observation, the status of which does not depend on the identification of the hypothesized mediators of the relationship.

Recently, Contrada, Wright, and Glass (1985), in considering the Houston/ Holmes debate, assessed a large sample of the relevant literature. They concluded that the method of measuring the Type A construct plays a large role in the determination of Type A/Type B differences in physiological responsivity and should not be ignored. Of the two most widely used measures, only the SI, and not the JAS has been consistently associated with the predicted greater reactivity of Type As. They point out that the uniqueness of the SI lies in its ability to detect ". . . hostility and vigorous speech stylistics" (p. 23), which are aspects of the Type A character ". . . most capable of discriminating CHD cases from noncases" (p. 23).

Finally, yet another view of the relationship between physiological factors and Type A behavior has been advanced by Krantz and Durel (1983). In a study of patients undergoing artery bypass surgery, Krantz, Arabian, Davia, and Parker (1982) found that even under general anesthesia, the intensity of SI-defined Type A behavior was positively correlated with magnitude of intraoperative increases in SBP. Similar results have been reported elsewhere in the literature (Kahn, Kornfeld, Frank, Heller, & Hoar, 1982). According to Krantz, Arabian, and co-workers (1982), these results suggest that there is a psychobiological substrate for Type A behavior, as increased cardiovascular responsiveness was observed under these conditions of minimal conscious mediation. Additional support for this view was found in several recent studies using beta-adrenergic medication. Schmeider, Friedrich, Neus, and Ruddel (1982) found that when sympathetic activity was attenuated with a beta-blocker (atenolol) over a 4-week period, this was correlated with a decrease in the intensity of Type A behavior (as assessed by the SI). Such a decrease in Type A behavior was not observed in a control group that received a diuretic over the same period. Krantz, Durel, and co-workers (1982) corroborated and extended these findings. They compared behavioral and psychophysiological responding among coronary patients who were either medicated or not medicated with the beta-blocking drug propranolol. Results indicated that the patients taking propranolol were lower in the intensity of their SI-defined Type A behavior than were the patients not taking the drug. These effects were not found among control patients. The propranolol patients also showed lower heart rate during a structured interview but did not differ in blood pressure from the other patients. The Type A features that were reduced in the propranolol patients were *speech stylistics* (loud/explosive speech, rapid accelerated speech, potential for hostility); however, the *content* of what the Type As said during the interview was unaffected by propranolol.

An explanation for these and other results was couched within a Schachterian model of emotions. In this view, the Type A pattern is the product of an interaction between cognitive and physiological elements, with speech stylistics reflecting underlying physiological responses. However, content aspects of the SI and scores on the JAS are more heavily influenced by cognitive-perceptual factors. It is hypothesized that the cognitive and physiological components produce the expression of Type A behavior through a mechanism involving feedback from peripheral sympathetic responses. The perception of, and cardiovascular response to, peripheral responses would encourage Type A stylistics; and conversely, the reduction of sympathetic responses by beta-blockers would reduce such stylistics. That atenolol, a beta-blocker with poor central nervous system penetration, reduced Type A behavior, supports this peripheral feedback view of Type A behavior.

Psychological Dimensions of the Type A Behavior Pattern

In this section research and theory on the psychological dimensions of the Type A behavior pattern will be reviewed. Our review will briefly examine the evidence relevant to the uncontrollability hypothesis of Type A behavior and then focus on recent evidence for the hostility component, which is thought to play an important role in the relationship between Type A behavior and CHD.

The idea that control is an important aspect of the Type A's intercourse with the environment (Glass, 1977), is the most popular and well-researched one in the psychological literature (Matthews, 1982). Briefly stated, this hypothesis suggests that Type As have an intense drive to succeed and to demonstrate control over their environment. In early research, the response patterns to uncontrollable failure by Type As and Bs were compared to evaluate the hypothesis (Krantz, Glass, & Snyder, 1974). This research showed that in response to experimentally induced failure, Type A individuals initially made more vigorous attempts to regain control than did Type Bs, but that following extended exposure to salient uncontrollablity they gave up and acted helpless (Krantz et al., 1974). Similarly, again during imposed and continuous failure, Brunson and Matthews (1981) showed that Type As used dysfunctional problem solving strategies and blamed themselves for their poor performance, whereas Type Bs continued to use adaptive strategies and attributed their failure to the difficulty of the task. Carver (1981) and Rhodewalt and Comer (1982) have also demonstrated that Type As are more threatened by loss of control than are Type Bs, and that they initially resist such threats by attempting to reestablish control.

Two experiments in our laboratory bear on the issue of controllability (Dyck, Moser, & Janisse, 1987). We focused on this variable because the hypothesized tendency to maintain and enhance self-esteem by controlling stressful aspects of their environment is considered basic to understanding the Type A syndrome. To date, most investigations of the control hypothesis have utilized indirect measures of perceived control and/or laboratory paradigms, however, we chose to study perceptions of control and causality using a more direct methodology and naturally occurring outcomes. In these experiments the subjects recalled past experiences involving competition and time pressure and provided ratings of vividness, perceived control for self, and perceived control for others in these situations. Type As recalled these experiences more vividly than did Type Bs. However, it was only in the recalled competitive situation that Type As felt themselves to be more in control than Type Bs. There were no differences between Type As and Bs in their perception of control for others in either situation . It would seem then that the Type A's perception of control is heightened by interpersonal competition situations, as differences did not emerge in the impersonal time pressure situation.

In a more general vein, we (Janisse, Dyck, & Malcolm, 1986) have found the Vando (1969) measure of stimulus intensity modulation (the reducer-augmenter dimension) to be positively related to both Type A and Speed and Impatience on the Jenkins Activity Survey. This supports the hypothesis that Type A individuals tend to enhance stimulus input, most likely (we believe) to better maintain control over their environment. In a factor analysis of several personality variables, these elements also made their presence felt in a separate "control" factor consisting of global Type A, stimulus intensity modulation, and speed and impatience.

Further comments on the importance of control have included a recent distinction between the desire for control and locus of control; that is, counterposing the desire to control outcomes versus beliefs or expectancies of control over outcomes (Dembroski, MacDougall, & Musante, 1984). These authors found a significant positive relationship between the desire to control and the Type A behavior pattern. Belief in control, however, was unrelated to the SI measure of Type A. Quite possibly, in discussing control and the Type A individual, it has been a mistake not to distinguish between the two aspects of control—desire and belief. Taken together, the motivational and cognitive/perceptual aspects of control likely interact with each other and situational variables to affect how Type As and Type Bs perceive their environment.

Following from the above, in a study of "real life" situations (Janisse, Yerama, & Dyck, 1987), Type A and Type B students made attributions for the outcome of a midterm examination in a university course. The type A students made more self-serving attributions than did the Type B students. That is, if they viewed their grade as a successful achievement, the Type As attributed this outcome to their own ability—more so than did Type Bs. On the other hand, when Type As viewed their grade as a failure, they attributed this outcome more to bad luck than did the Type B subjects. In general, Type As more so than Type Bs, tended to attribute success to internal, stable causes and failure to external, unstable causes. It should be noted that the subjects labeled their performance after they had viewed their examination scores in the context of the class distribution of marks. Thus there was ample opportunity for the subjects to evaluate their performance relative to others. The results of Dyck and colleagues (1987) and Janisse and colleagues (1987) confirm the hypothesis that, not only are Type As concerned with maintaining control and enhancing their self-esteem (through self-serving attributions)—Strube (1985), has reached a similar conclusion—their own perceptions of control may be rooted in social comparison processes; that is, control is defined relative to others. Recall that in Dyck and colleagues (1987), Type As differed from Type Bs in attributing to themselves greater control only in competitive situations, and that in Janisse and colleagues (1987) class grades, averages, etc. were posted for all students to see.

The manner in which social comparison processes impact on perceptions of control was revealed in a recent study utilizing a judgment of contingency paradigm (Moser & Dyck, 1987). In the context of a button pressing task, Type A and Type B subjects were asked to judge how much control they (self) or an experimental confederate (other) had in producing a frequently occurring but noncontingent outcome (i.e., a green light appeared on 50% of the trials independent of button presses). The results indicated that although

Type As and Bs did not differ on global judgments of control, Type As reported that the desirable outcome (green light) was more frequent for the confederate than it was for themselves, independent of whether or not a press had been made. Type Bs, on the other hand, saw themselves rewarded just as frequently as the confederate. These results imply that Type As may perceive environmental contingencies of reward as being more lenient for others than for themselves. Given this perception, it follows that Type As conclude that they must strive harder relative to others to get the things that they want. It is also possible that the perception of differential contingencies of reinforcement for self and others by Type As plays a role in fostering the development of hostility and anger among Type As by creating the conditions for perceived injustice and/or jealousy. It is to the recent evidence on the hostility component of the Type A behavior pattern that we now direct our attention.

As noted previously, it has been suggested that the anger and hostility component of Type A is particularly relevant to the prediction of CHD (e.g., Matthews et al., 1977) and researchers have increasingly become interested in this component. Early attempts to validate the hostility component independent of the Type A assessment procedure used self-report measures of anger and hostility with mixed results (e.g., Chesney, Black, Chadwick, & Rosenman, 1981; Dimsdale, Hackett, Block, & Hutter, 1978; Francis, 1981; Zurawski & Houston, 1983). In retrospect, the inconsistent results derive from a failure to control social desirability variables. More specifically, it appears that Type As will endorse more hostile self-descriptors than will Type Bs only when the adjectives are socially acceptable, such as those that also have achievement connotations (Herman, Blumenthal, Black, & Chesney, 1981). Thus, the use of self-report measures that rely solely on "controlled" forms of processing are subject to a social desirability bias, and therefore of limited utility in assessing A/B differences. (An example of just such a problem, resulting in two similar studies finding dissimilar results, is described in a paper by Williams [in press].)

Given the preceding, we believe paradigms that to some extent reflect "automatic" processing (e.g., incidental recall) have proven more promising in detecting A/B differences. For example, in a recent adaptation of a self-referent recall paradigm used in depression research (Kuiper & Derry, 1982), it was found that self-referent recall for endorsed hostile words was greater among Type As than among Type Bs following noncontingent failure (Moser & Dyck, 1987) and provocation (Yuen, Janisse, & Dyck, 1987). These effects were not observed in nonstimulated controls. Further, on the basis of a median split on the number of hostile words endorsed, it was found that hostile self-referent ratings following provocation led to increased aggression, as measured by the endorsement of hostile letters given to the provocative confederate (Yuen et al., 1987). Thus, following noncontingent failure and provocation Type As process hostility information more efficiently than do Type Bs. Further, the ease with which individuals process hostility information predicts behavioral aggression. Interestingly, in the Yuen and co-workers study, no differences in aggression were observed between Type As and Bs.

Cognitive and imaginal procedures have also been found to be useful in identifying A/B differences in hostility (e.g., Baker, Hastings, & Hart, 1984; Janisse, Edguer, & Dyck, 1986). For example, Janisse and co-workers (1986) were able to produce A/B differences in ratings of anger and heart rate, particularly among subjects scoring above the median on anger expression (Spielberger et al., 1985) by having subjects recall and imagine angry experiences or by employing a Velten (1968) procedure utilizing appropriate self-referent statements. It was found that Type As high on anger expressiveness reported lower ratings of self-control than did Type As low in anger expressiveness, thereby supporting the hypothesized link between loss of control in Type As and angry reactions to provocative stimuli.

Finally, a number of studies have recently investigated the relation between Type A behavior and laboratory aggression. Some of these investigations have reported increased hostile aggression by Type As following frustration (Strube et al., 1984) and provocation (Check & Dyck, 1986), whereas other investigations have not found A/B differences. For example, in a recent examination of the role of provocation and possible retaliation on aggression and physiological reactions, Edguer (1987) found no A/B differences in aggression. On the other hand, A/B differences in heart rate and blood pressure were observed and these were the largest when subjects were both provoked and led to expect retaliation. This latter result agrees with a number of studies that have shown A/B differences in physiological reactions to provocative, frustrative, or challenging circumstances (Dembroski et al., 1978; Dembroski, MacDougall, Herd, & Shields, 1979; Diamond et al., 1984; Glass & Carver, 1980).

The evidence from the personality and "psychological" research areas seems to point consistently to control as a key factor in the behavior of the Type A. How this comes about developmentally and how it is activated in specific situations are areas that are still in need of investigation. In the following section we offer some guidelines to future research that will integrate the role of physiological and psychological variables in CHD.

Conclusion

Research on the physiological mediation of Type A emphasizes the importance of sympathetic reactivity and, importantly, the interpretation of peripheral feedback in exacerbating Type A stylistics. On the other hand, research with psychological mediators of Type A behavior emphasizes the role of control and situationally specific stressors as eliciting variables. This research also identifies the anger/hostility component as being particularly important to the prediction of CHD risk. However, it is not known how physiological mediation interacts with the psychological aspects to produce the expression of Type A behavior; particularly the anger/hostility component. Three questions emerge: 1) Does the heightened physiological reactivity exhibited by Type As in challenging situations contribute to ego threat and attempts to regain control in a hostile and aggressive manner? Or 2) Do Type As engender the challenges that they then respond to with increased cardiovascular activity? And 3), given the contention of Markus (1977) that schemas often create the reality they anticipate together with the recent observation of A/B differences in hostility schemata, is it possible that Type As with hostility schemata may be more likely to a) interpret interpersonal messages as hostile, b) send communications that are more hostile than necessary, and c) demonstrate an exaggerated cardiovascular response in such "created" situations? (cf. Smith & Rhodewalt, 1986.) Further, an intriguing but as yet unanswered possibility is that not all Type As are equally dependent on situational factors (psychological) for the elicitation of the Type A behavior pattern. If this is so, a corollary question is, are Type As with varying thresholds of environmental challenge equally at risk for CHD? In this regard, it would be interesting to test the hypothesis that those Type As with lower thresholds for hostility would be more susceptible to CHD. At the extreme may be those Type As who engender challenges and exhibit increased cardiovascular activity in its absence!

Acknowledgments.   Portions of this chapter were written while Dr. Janisse was Visiting Professor of the Sonderforschungbereich 99, Department of Psychology, University of Konstanz, Konstanz, West Germany. He would like to thank Dr. Robert Freeman and Dr. Michael Schluroff for making their facilities available. Some research described herein was supported by a grant to Dr. Dyck from the University of Manitoba/SSHRCC Fund Committee.

References

Baker, L.J., Hastings, J.E., & Hart, J.D. (1984). Enhanced psychophysiological responses of Type A coronary patients during Type A-relevant imagery. *Journal of Behavioral Medicine, 7*, 287–306.

Brunson, B.I., & Matthews, K.A. (1981). The Type A coronary-prone behavior pattern: An analysis of performance strategies, affect, and attributing during failure. *Journal of Personality and Social Psychology, 40*, 916–918.

Carruthers, M.E. (1969). Aggression and atheroma. *Lancet, 2*, 1170.

Carver, C.S. (1981). Perceived coersion, resistance to persuasion, and the Type A behavior pattern. *Journal of Research in Personality, 19*, 467–481.

Carver, C.S., Coleman, A.E., & Glass, D.C. (1976). The coronary prone behavior pattern and the suppression of fatigue on a treadmill test. *Journal of Personality and Social Psychology, 33*, 460–466.

Carver, C.S., & Glass, D.C. (1978). Coronary-prone behavior pattern and interpersonal aggression. *Journal of Personality and Social Psychology, 36*, 361–366.

Check, J., & Dyck, D.G. (1986). Hostile aggression and Type A behavior. *Personality and Individual Differences*, 7, 819–827.

Chesney, M.A., Black, G.W., Chadwick, J.H., & Rosenman, R.H. (1981). Psychological correlates of coronary-prone behavior. *Journal of Behavioral Medicine*, 4, 217–230.

Contrada, R.J., Wright, R.A., & Glass, D.C. (1985). Psychophysiologic correlates of Type A behavior: Comments on Houston (1983) and Holmes (1983). *Journal of Research in Personality*, 19, 12–30.

Corse, C.D., Manuck, S.B., Cantwell, J.D., Giordani, B., & Matthews, K.A. (1982). Coronary prone behavior pattern and cardiovascular response in persons with and without coronary heart disease. *Psychosomatic Medicine*, 44, 449–459.

Dembroski, T.M., MacDougall, J.M., Herd, J.A., & Shields, J.L. (1979). Effect of level of challenge on pressor and heart rate responses in Type A and Type B subjects. *Journal of Applied Social Psychology*, 9, 209–228.

Dembroski, T.M., MacDougall, J.M., & Musante, L. (1984). Desirability of control versus locus of control: Relationship to paralinguistics in the Type A interview. *Health Psychology*, 3, 15–26.

Dembroski, T.M., MacDougall, J.M., Shields, J.L., Petillo, V., & Lushene, R. (1978). Components of the Type A coronary-prone behavior pattern and cardiovascular response to psychomotor challenge. *Journal of Behavioral Medicine*, 1, 159–176.

Dembroski, T.M., Weiss, S.M., Shields, J.L., Haynes, S., & Feinleib, M. (Eds.) (1978). *Coronary-prone behavior*. New York: Springer-Verlag.

Diamond, E.L., Schneider, N., Schwartz, D., Smith, J.C., Vorp, R., & Pasin, R.D. (1984). Harassment, hostility and Type A as determinants of cardiovascular reactivity during competition. *Journal of Behavioral Medicine*, 7, 171–189.

Dimsdale, J.E., Hackett, T.P., Block, P.C., & Hutter, A.M. (1978). Emotional correlates of the Type A behavior pattern. *Psychosomatic Medicine*, 40, 580–583.

Dyck, D.G., Moser, C.G., & Janisse, M.P. (1987). Type A behavior and situation specific perceptions of control. *Psychological Reports*, 60, 991–999.

Edguer, N. (1987). *Type A behavior and aggression: Provocation, conflict and physiological responsivity in the Buss teacher-learner paradigm*. Unpublished doctoral dissertation, University of Manitoba, Winnipeg, Canada.

Francis, K. (1981). Perceptions of hostility, anxiety and depression in subjects exhibiting the coronary-prone behavior pattern. *Journal of Psychiatric Research*, 16, 183–190.

Friedman, M. (1969). *Pathogenesis of coronary heart disease*. New York: McGraw-Hill.

Friedman, M., Byers, S.O., Diamont, J., & Rosenman, R.H. (1975). Plasma catecholamic response of coronary-prone subjects (Type A) to a specific challenge. *Metabolism*, 24, 205.

Friedman, M., & Rosenman, R.H. (1974). *Type A behavior and your heart*. New York: Knopf.

Glass, D.C. (1977). *Behavior patterns, stress and coronary disease*. Hillsdale, NJ: Lawrence Erlbaum Associates.

Glass, D.C., & Carver, C.S. (1980). Helplessness and the coronary-prone personality. In J. Garber and M.E.P. Seligman (Eds.), *Human helplessness* (pp. 223–243). New York: Academic Press.

Goldband, S. (1980). Stimulus specificity of physiological response to stress and the coronary-prone behavior pattern. *Journal of Personality and Social Psychology*, 39, 670–679.

Hames, C.G., Lightman, M.A., & McDonough, J.T. (1965). Postexercise plasma and urinary norepinephrine and epinephrine levels among high school and low social class males and subjects with non-acute coronary heart disease. *Circulation (Supplement III)*, *32*, 105.

Herman, S., Blumenthal, J.A., Black, G.M., & Chesney, M.A. (1981). Self-ratings of Type A (Coronary-prone) adults. Do Type A's know they are Type A's? *Psychosomatic Medicine*, *43*, 405–414.

Holmes, D.S. (1983). An alternative perspective concerning the differential psychophysiological responsivity of persons with the Type A and Type B behavior patterns. *Journal of Research in Personality*, *17*, 40–47.

Houston, B.K. (1983). Physiological responsivity and the Type A behavior pattern. *Journal of Research in Personality*, *17*, 22–39.

Janisse, M.P., Dyck, D.G., & Malcolm, A.T. (1986). Personality, control, and the Type A behavior pattern. Unpublished manuscript, University of Manitoba, Winnipeg, Canada.

Janisse, M.P., Edguer, N., & Dyck, D.G. (1986). Type A behavior, anger expression and reactions to anger imagery. *Motivation and Emotion*, *8*, 373–388.

Janisse, M.P., Yerama, C., & Dyck, D.G. (1987). Type A behavior and the processing of causal attributions in laboratory and naturally occurring settings. Manuscript under review, University of Manitoba, Winnipeg, Canada.

Jenkins, C.D., Zyzanski, S.T., & Rosenman, R.H. (1971). Progress toward a validation of a computer-scored test for the Type A coronary-prone behavior pattern. *Psychosomatic Medicine*, *33*, 193–202.

Kahn, J.P., Kornfeld, D.S., Frank, K.A., Heller, S.S., & Hoar, P.F. (1982). Type A behavior and blood pressure during coronary bypass surgery. *Psychosomatic Medicine*, *42*, 407–414.

Krantz, D.S., Arabian, J.M., Davia, J.E., & Parker, J.S. (1982). Type A behavior and coronary artery bypass surgery: Intraoperative blood pressure and perioperative complication. *Psychosomatic Medicine*, *44*, 273–294.

Krantz, D.S., & Durel, L.A. (1983). Psychobiological substrates of the Type A behavior pattern. *Journal of Health Psychology*, *2*, 393–411.

Krantz, D.S., Durel, L.A., Davia, J.E., Shaffer, R.T., Arabian, J.M., Dembroski, T.M., & MacDougall, J.M. (1982). Propranolol medication among coronary patients: Relationship to Type A behavior and cardiovascular response. *Journal of Human Stress*, *8*, 4–12.

Krantz, D.S., Glass, D.C., & Snyder, M.L. (1974). Helplessness, stress level, and the coronary-prone behavior pattern. *Journal of Experimental Social Psychology*, *10*, 284–300.

Kuiper, N.A., & Derry, P.A. (1982). Depressed and nondepressed content self-reference in mild depressives. *Journal of Personality*, *50*, 67–79.

Malcolm, A.T., Janisse, M.P., & Dyck, D.G. (1984). Type A behavior, heart rate and pupillary response: Effects of cold pressor and ego threat. *Journal of Psychosomatic Research*, *28*, 27–34.

Markus, H. (1977). Self-schemata and processing information about the self. *Journal of Personality and Social Psychology*, *35*, 63–78.

Matthews, K.A. (1982). Psychological perspectives on the Type A behavior pattern. *Psychological Bulletin*, *91*, 293–323.

Matthews, K.A., Glass, D.C., Rosenman, R.H., & Bortner, R.W. (1977). Competitive drive, pattern A, and coronary heart disease: A further analysis of some data from the collaborative group study. *Journal of Chronic Diseases*, *30*, 489–498.

Moser, C.G., & Dyck, D.G. (1987). Type A behavior and judgments of control for self and others. Manuscript under review, University of Manitoba, Winnipeg, Canada.

Nestle, P.J., Verghese, A., & Lovell, R.R. (1967). Catecholamine secretion and sympathetic nervous system responses to emotion in men with and without angina pectoris. *American Heart Journal, 73*, 227.

Pittner, M.S., & Houston, B.K. (1980). Response to stress, cognitive coping strategies, and the Type A behavior pattern. *Journal of Personality and Social Psychology, 39*, 147–157.

Rhodewalt, F., & Comer, R. (1982). Coronary-prone behavior and the experience of reactance in the choice elimination paradigm. *Personality and Social Psychology Bulletin, 8*, 1521–158.

Rosenman, R.H., Brand, R.J., Jenkins, C.D., Friedman, M., Strauss, R., & Wurm, M. (1975). Coronary heart disease in the Western Collaborative Heart Study: Final follow-up experience of 8 1/2 years. *Journal of the American Medical Association, 232*, 872–877.

Rosenman, R.H., Friedman, M., Straus, R., Wurm, M., Kositchek, R., Hahn, W., & Werthessen, N.T. (1964). A predictive study of coronary heart disease. *Journal of the American Medical Association, 189*, 103–110.

Rosenman, R.H., Rahe, R.H., Borhani, N.D., & Feinleib, M. (1976). Heritability of personality and behavior pattern. *Acta Geveticae Medicae et Gemellologiae, 25*, 221–224.

Schmeider, R., Friedrich, G., Neus, J., & Ruddel, J. (1982). Effect of B-blockers on Type A coronary-prone behavior. *Psychosomatic Medicine, 44*, 129–130.

Smith, T.W., & Rhodewalt, F. (1986). On states, traits and processes: A transactional alternative to the individual difference assumptions in Type A behavior and physiological reactivity. *Journal of Research in Personality, 20*, 229–251.

Spielberger, C.D., Johnson, E., Russell, S., Crane, R.S., Jacobs, G., & Worden, T.I. (1985). The experience and expression of anger: Construction and validation of an anger expression scale. In M.A. Chesney and R.H. Rosenman (Eds.), *Anger and hostility in cardiovascular and behavioral disorders* (pp. 5–29). New York: Hemisphere/McGraw-Hill.

Strube, M.J. (1985). Attributional style and the Type A coronary-prone behavior pattern. *Journal of Personality and Social Psychology, 49*, 500–509.

Strube, M.J. (1987). A self-appraisal model of the Type A behavior pattern. In R. Hogan and W. Jones (Eds.), *Perspectives in personality: Theory, measurement and interpersonal dynamics* (pp.). Greenwich, CT: JAI Press.

Strube, M.J., Turner, C.W., Cerro, D., Stevens, J., & Hinchey, F. (1984). Interpersonal aggression and the Type A coronary-prone behavior pattern: A theoretical distinction and practical implications. *Journal of Personality and Social Psychology, 47*, 829–847.

Vando, A. (1969). *A personality dimension related to pain tolerance.* Unpublished doctoral dissertation, Columbia University, New York.

Velten, E. (1968). A laboratory test for the induction of mood states. *Behavior Research and Therapy, 6*, 437–482.

Weiss, J.M., Stone, E.A., & Harrell, N. (1970). Coping behavior and brain epinephrine in rats. *Journal of Comparative and Physiological Psychology, 72*, 153–160.

Williams, R.B. Jr. (in press). Coronary-prone behavior: The emerging role of the hostility complex. In B.K. Houston and C.R. Snyder (Eds.), *Type A behavior pattern: Current trends and future directions.* New York: John Wiley & Sons.

Yuen, S., Janisse, M.P., & Dyck, D.G. (1987). Hostile self-schemata, hostile aggression and the Jenkins Activity Survey measure of Type A behavior. Unpublished manuscript, University of Manitoba, Winnipeg, Canada.

Zurawski, R.M., & Houston, B.K. (1983). The Jenkins Activity Survey measure of Type-A and frustration induced anger. *Motivation and Emotion, 7,* 301–312.

4

Sensation Seeking, Risk Taking, and Health

Marvin Zuckerman

In this chapter, Zuckerman concentrates on the literature pertaining to the concept of risk taking/sensation seeking as it relates to health concerns. After discussing the data on hypertension and sensation seekers—much of it showing a seemingly more dangerous *elevated* blood pressure in low scorers on the sensation seeking scale—he describes similar counter-intuitive results for users of nicotine, alcohol, and other drugs. He analyzes the consistent finding that risk takers, along with smokers, drinkers, and drug users have lower blood pressure than their more abstemious counterparts. A large section of the chapter is devoted to smoking, ". . . a major risk factor, not only for lung cancer, but for other types of cancer and cardiovascular disease as well." He reviews the changes in the demographics of smoking during the last 15 to 20 years, based on data he gathered in 1970 and in 1986. The association between smoking and the sensation seeking dimension is a complex one; although every group seems to be smoking less since 1970, the high sensation seeker is still the greater user of nicotine. The data are moderated by such factors as gender, amount smoked, time since beginning to smoke, and amount of smoke inhaled. It is of note that level of sensation seeking appears to be unrelated to success in quitting or attempts to quit. Also explored in this chapter are the reasons for smoking; the evidence indicates that high sensation seekers smoke both to increase arousal and, at times, to decrease negatively toned arousal. This was discovered through the development of a new smoking questionnaire, described in the chapter, which yields three major factors: relaxation or boredom, attention-concentration, and negative emotional arousal. The concluding section of the chapter offers some insightful thoughts and data on personality and health that are provocative and provide direction for future research.

—Editor

The last decade in America might be called "the age of hypochondria" because of the preoccupation with personal health. Americans are concerned about their diets, exercise, and all kinds of cancerogenic threats in smoking and other environmental pollutants. Health-food shops and exercise parlors, stocked with devices resembling medieval torture instruments, are found everywhere. It is difficult to make one's way down a supermarket aisle because of all the people reading the small print listing the ingredients in foods. The antismokers are in the ascendancy and crowding the smokers into increasingly smaller and more isolated spaces. In the middle of all of this the AIDS epidemic arrived and is reputed to be changing the sex habits of America in what can be termed a "counterrevolution" to the sexual revolution of the 1970s.

All of this is not to deprecate the concerns over health, but to point out the changing perceptions of risk. In an age when people are actually living longer than previous generations, they perceive greater threats to their health. Much of our health fate is probably determined by genetically regulated vulnerabilities, but it is reasonable to deal as well as we can with the behavioral and environmental risk factors that are under our control. Preventive medicine is in vogue because of the failure to devise specific cures for serious diseases such as cancer and AIDs.

Personality traits provide constructs to explain the types of risk-taking behaviors that threaten health and well-being. But at a more basic level, personality may be involved in health because of differences in biological vulnerabilities relevant to specific health problems. I believe this may be the case for the link between sensation seeking and hypertension. Although no studies have been done on the sensation-seeking tendencies in heart disorders and cancer, there is a connection between sensation seeking and smoking, and smoking is one of the high risk factors involved in these disorders. Whereas many persons have quit smoking without benefit of professional help, psychological programs to aid smokers in their efforts to quit have failed, perhaps because of the disregard for individual differences in the reasons for smoking. A study will be reported that investigated the relation between personality and the situational control of smoking. Cognitive differences between high and low sensation seekers in risk appraisal were also studied.

Hypertension

Our first hint of a relationship between sensation seeking and hypertension came from some serendipitous findings from a study of drug effects on high and low sensation seekers. Carrol, Zuckerman, and Vogel (1982) selected male medical students scoring in the upper and lower deciles on the Total score of the Sensation Seeking Scale form V (SSSV) (Zuckerman, 1979a) as subjects. It is important to note that these were extreme scorers on the SSS. Because they were to be given both stimulant (amphetamine) and depressant (diazepam) drugs during the experimental sessions, all potential subjects were screened by a medical examination including a diagnostic interview. The medical examination was repeated after the three seessions of the experiment to insure that there were no residual effects. Blood pressure readings were taken by the examining physician who did both exams. During the experimental sessions blood pressure readings were taken by a nurse before and after the administration of drugs or placebo.

Four potential subjects were excluded from the experiment because of a personal history of hypertension; all were low sensation seekers. None of the high sensation seekers were excluded for any medical reason. Despite this screening of hypertensives, the systolic blood pressures recorded by the physician for the remaining low sensation seekers, both in the exam before ($M = 136$mm Hg) and after ($M = 138$mm Hg) the experiment, were significantly higher than those of the high sensation seekers (126mm Hg on both occasions). Curiously, the high and low sensation seekers did not differ significantly on the systolic blood pressures recorded by the nurse before and after the three experimental sessions. The effect might have been written off as a specific effect produced by the examining physician, except for some additional findings from the medical case history. Nine of the 16 (56%) low sensation seeking subjects accepted in the study reported having parents or immediate relatives with a history of cardiovascular diseases including hypertension, myocardial infarction, and cerebral vascular accident, whereas only 3 of the 16 (19%) of the high sensation seeking students reported this kind of family history. The difference in these proportions was significant. The examining physician was blind as to the sensation seeking scores of the subjects.

A greater proportion of the high sensation seeking than low sensation seeking students admitted to smoking tobacco and marijuana, using alcohol, and a variety of illegal drugs. Six of the 16 (38%) low sensation seekers abstained from all drugs including alcohol and tobacco. Not one of the high sensation seekers reported this kind of substance-free history. Conversely, 88% of the high and only 13% of the low sensation seekers used marijuana, and 44% of the high sensation seekers and none of the low reported using illegal drugs other than maijuana. Clearly, the high sensation seekers were ingesting many things that could raise their blood pressures, but it was the "clean living" lows who showed higher blood pressure readings during the physical examinations.

In two subsequent studies conducted in our laboratory we could not find significant differences in the blood pressure of high and low sensation seekers using an automatically inflated sphygmomanometer and recorder. For instance, a study by Litle (1986) that examined differences between highs and lows in an experiment using a horror film as a stressor found systolic BP differences ranging from 2mm Hg at baseline to 6mm Hg at one of the stress periods. None of these differences were significant, although the low sensation seekers always had the higher BPs.

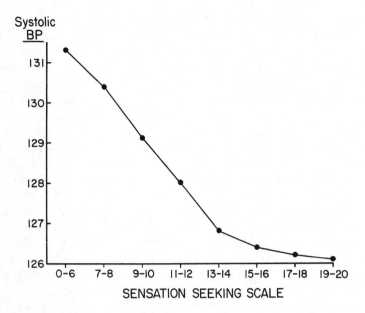

Figure 4.1. Means levels of systolic blood pressure at different ranges of sensation seeking scores. Based on unpublished data from a study by von Knorring, Oreland, and Winblad (1984).

A significant relationship between systolic blood pressure and sensation seeking emerged from a large study of over 1,000 Swedish male army recruits (von Knorring, Oreland, & Winblad, 1984). Blood pressures were taken during a physical exam. Figure 4.1 shows the mean systolic BPs at eight class intervals of scores on the SSSV. The relationship was a significant one ($p < .001$) even though the range of systolic blood pressure from the highest to the lowest category was only 5mm Hg. Actually, the average and high scorers had systolic blood pressures close to the average for the population (about 128mm Hg). It was only the lowest 9% of sensation seekers (scores 0 to 6) who showed a mean elevation of blood pressure outside of the normal range and even this mean of 131.3 was not in the clinical range defining borderline hypertension (above 140).

The high sensation seekers tended to have low levels of the enzyme monoamine oxidase (MAO) and subjects with such low levels of MAO had indications of heavy drinking or even alcoholism in their histories, including blackouts and signs of dependence. They were also more likely to be regular cigarette smokers, cannabis abusers, and glue sniffers. As in the Carrol and co-workers (1982) study, the group with habits likely to promote hypertension was paradoxically normal in blood pressure, whereas the low sensation seeking subjects, who rarely or never smoked or drank and almost never used dangerous drugs, showed significant elevations in blood pressure.

Although not a recommendation of drinking, smoking, and drug use for health, these results suggest that the personality factor of sensation seeking and its associated biological traits are more crucial in vulnerability to hypertension than the specific effects of alcohol, smoking, or drug abuse.

Schalling and Svensson (1984) studied personality traits related to blood pressure in Swedish army recruits from the Stockholm area. Although none of these subjects had been diagnosed as hypertensive, routine blood pressure readings during their physical examination revealed one group of subjects with systolic BP in the borderline hypertensive range (above 146mm Hg) and another group in the hypotensive range (systolic BP 100–106mm Hg). A comparison group of normotensives (with systolic BP in the range 124–131) were also studied. Significant differences were found between hypertensives and normotensives on scales of anxiety, tension, and neuroticism, and a scale labeled "Inhibition of Aggression;" the hypertensives were higher than normotensives on these scales. Hypotensives tended to be higher than hypertensives and normotensives on the scale "Monotony Avoidance," a Swedish version of the Sensation Seeking Scale. The picture of the hypertensive as someone who is anxious and inhibits or suppresses rage or anger and is nonassertive is consistent with Alexander's (1939) early description of the hypertensive personality, but contrary to the Type-A concept of a person who is openly aggressive, competitive, assertive, and impatient.

It is my view that relationships between personality and psychophysiology are mediated by individual differences in biochemical traits. What is the biochemical trait that might link sensation seeking, anxiety, and suppression of anger to elevated blood pressure? Both peripheral and central noradrengeric activity has been linked to regulation of blood pressure. The urinary metabolite of norepinephrine, 3-methoxy-4 hydroxyphenylglycol, or MHPG, is correlated positively with systolic BP in depressed and normal and hypertensive patients (Potter, Muscettola, & Goodwin, 1983). Drugs, such as clonidine, morphine, benzodiazepines, and tricyclic antidepressants, which reduce noradrenergic activity in the locus ceruleus, also lower blood pressure and reduce anxiety and panic (Charney & Heninger, 1986). Yohimbine, a drug that increases noradrenergic activity in the locus ceruleus by blocking the negative feedback mechanism, also results in increases in MHPG, systolic BP, and anxiety, particularly in panic-prone patients and agoraphobics. The positive association between very high levels of noradrenergic activity and anxiety trait is apparent in these data. But what of sensation seeking?

A significant negative correlation was found between noradrenaline in the cerebrospinal fluid and sensation seeking in a study by Ballenger and co-workers (1983). The direction of the correlation is consistent with negative correlations found between dopamine-beta-hydroxylase (DBH), the enzyme that converts dopamine to noradrenaline in the noradrenaline neuron, and sensation seeking in this study (Ballenger et al., 1983) as well as studies by Umberkoman-Wiita, Vogel, and Wiita (1981) and Kulcsár, Kutor, and Arató (1984). If DBH is low then less dopamine will be converted to noradrenaline. At any rate, these correlational data are consistent with the higher blood pressure found in low sensation seekers because they have relatively higher levels of CSF noradrenaline than the highs. According to the optimal level of catecholamine systems theory (Zuckerman, 1984), positive affect emerges at some intermediate level of catecholamine activity. High sensation seekers are below this level and low sensation seekers are at or above this level while in an unstimulated state or monotonous environment. Highs will seek activities that stimulate catecholamine systems, whereas lows will avoid such stimulation because any increase of catecholamine systems activity pushes them into a range characterized by sympathetic system overarousal and anxiety.

Smoking

Changes in the Population and Relationships with Sensation Seeking

Smoking has been implicated as a major health risk factor, not only for lung cancer, but for other types of cancer and cardiovascular disease as well. In the United States the government and medical profession have waged a campaign to reduce smoking and statistics show that it has been successful in reducing the proportion of the smoking population. Social influence may certainly affect the relationship between basic personality traits and their behavioral expressions. The relationship between smoking and sensation seeking trait was studied at the University of Delaware in the early 1970s and again in 1986. Table 4.1 shows the proportions of low, medium, and high sensation seekers reporting current or past smoking experience. In 1970, 81% of high and 42% of low sensation seeking college women had some smoking experience, but in 1986 only 46% of the highs and 25% of the lows ever smoked. Among males in 1970, there was no relationship between any smoking and sensation seeking because the great majority in both groups smoked at least occasionally. But if we limit the smokers category to those smoking at least every day then two thirds of the highs and only one quarter of the lows turn out to have been habitual smokers. Most of the low sensation

Table 4.1. Percentages of Smokers (Past or Current) in Ranges of Sensation Seeking: 1970–1972 Compared with 1986

SS Range	Males		Females	
	High	Low	High	Low
1970	72	90	81	42
1986	34	15	48	25

	High	Medium	Low
1972	67	47	18
1986	34	24	15

seeking males were only occasional smokers, probably only in social settings. In 1972, two thirds of the high males had smoking experience, but in 1986 that proportion was halved. The proportion of medium sensation seekers in 1986 was also about half of that found in 1972, but there was little change in the already low proportion of low sensation seekers smoking from 1972 to 1986. Sensation seeking still has a significant relationship to smoking but there has been a marked reduction in smoking, particularly in medium and high sensation seekers.

The current data on smoking incidence and sensation seeking is based on 1,071 college students at the University of Delaware who took both the SSSV and a smoking questionnaire that contained questions about smoking habits. Only 14% of the sample were current smokers; another 18% were former smokers, and 68% had never smoked. More than twice as many females are current smokers than males (18% versus 7%), but about the same proportions of both sexes are past smokers (17% and 19%). Table 4.2 shows the sex difference, which was significant.

Combining the sexes and comparing the proportions of low, medium, and high sensation seekers never smoking, previously smoking, and currently smoking yields a significant difference (Table 4.3). The difference is also significant for males ($\chi^2 = 13.93$, $p < .01$) and females ($\chi^2 = 37.74$, $p < .001$) considered separately. More than twice as many high sensation seekers are current smokers (20%) as low sensation seekers (9%), and nearly twice as many high sensation seekers (23%) as low sensation seekers (13%) are

Table 4.2. Percentages of Males and Females in Three Smoking Status Categories

| | n | Smoking Status % | | |
		Never	Past	Current
Males	422	76	17	7
Females	649	63	19	18
All Ss	1071	68	18	14

$\chi^2 = 28.34$ (df $= 2$), $p < .001$

Table 4.3. Percentages of High, Medium, and Low Sensation Seekers in Three Smoking Status Categories

| SS | n | Smoking Status % | | |
		Never	Past	Current
High	360	57	23	20
Medium	349	68	20	12
Low	362	78	13	9

$\chi^2 = 40.10$ (df $= 2$), $p < .001$

Table 4.4. Sensation Seeking and the Smoking Habit

SS	n	How many years a smoker? %		Smoke in a day? %		How much inhale? %		Tried to quit? %		
		0–2	3≥	<1/2	≥1/2 pack	Never-Few	Most Puffs	No	Once	2X≥
High	85	66	34	66	34	19	81	28	36	36
Medium	45	78	22	84	16	44	56	33	44	23
Low	36	86	14	75	25	31	69	40	40	20

$\chi^2 = 5.97$ (df = 2) $p = .06$ $\chi^2 = 5.28, p<.10$ $\chi^2 = 13.07, p<.01$ $\chi^2 = 4.60$ (df = 4)

former smokers who have quit. More than three quarters (75%) of the low sensation seekers have never smoked compared with 57% of the highs.

More specific questions were asked about the smoking habit and its history (Table 4.4). When subjects were divided into those who had smoked only 2 years or less and those who had smoked 3 years or more, a greater proportion of the highs apparently started smoking earlier (all subjects were in the same age range). Most subjects were not heavy smokers. Almost three quarters (73%) of the subjects claimed they smoked less than half a pack per day. There was a tendency for a greater proportion of high sensation seekers to smoke a half pack or more per day but this was not significant ($p < .10$). However, there was a significant tendency for a greater proportion of high sensation seekers (81%) to report that they inhaled on almost every puff, as compared to medium (56%) or low (69%) sensation seekers. Subjects were asked if they had ever tried to quit smoking and how many times they tried. The differences in proportions of high, medium, and low sensation seekers who never tried and those who tried at least once was not significant whether we compared present smokers only or past and present smokers combined. A study by Zuckerman and Neeb (1980) compared SSS scores of past and present smokers and found no significant differences. Apparently, sensation seeking is not related to the motivation to quit smoking or the success in quitting smoking among those who try.

Two additional questions dealt with the cognitive appraisal of smoking risk (Table 4.5). Zuckerman (1979b) explored the risk evaluations of high and low sensation seekers on a variety of activities involving physical, social, or legal punishment risk. Sensation seeking scores on the Total scale correlated negatively and significantly with all three kinds of risk appraisal: high sensation seekers regarded these activities as less risky than did the lows. If a similar kind of difference in risk appraisal existed in regard to smoking, it might explain the greater smoking tendency among high sensation seekers. We therefore included a question in the smoking questionnaire that asked: "How great a health risk is smoking?" The subjects could respond "very small," "small," "moderate," "great," or "very great." As can be seen in Table 4.5, about half of these smoking subjects consider smoking a "very

Table 4.5. Sensation Seeking and Cognitive Estimates of Risk in Smoking

SS	n	How Great a Health Risk Is Smoking? %			What % of Heavy Smokers Develop Lung Cancer?		
		Small-Mod	Great	Very Great	5–20%	35%	50%
High	85	14	35	51	19	24	60
Medium	42	19	29	52	12	39	49
Low	37	24	22	54	27	24	49
All	164	18	30	52	19	27	54

$\chi^2 = 3.25$ (df = 4) p N.S. $\chi^2 = 6.35$ (df = 4) $p < .10$

great" health hazard and another 30% consider it a "great" risk. The relationship between the risk appraisal and sensation seeking was not significant. However, when the data were analyzed separately for current and past smokers there was a marked discrepancy in the responses of the low sensation seekers. Among past smokers, 78% of the low sensation seekers regarded smoking as a "very great" health risk, but among the current smokers only 32% of the low sensation seekers regarded smoking as this much of a health hazard. A similar discrepancy in responses of low sensation seekers as a function of whether or not they were currently smoking was found for the next question as well.

A second question asked was: "What percentage of heavy smokers do you think will develop lung cancer?" The response options were 5%, 10%, 20%, 35%, and 50%. More than half of the subjects (54%) chose the maximum risk value of 50%, a marked exaggeration of the actual risk which is about 20%. When past and current smokers are grouped together the relationship between the estimated risk and sensation seeking was not significant ($p < .10$). When past and current smokers were separated and two separate analyses were done of the relationship between risk appraisal and sensation seeking, the relationship was significant in the current smokers but not in the past smokers. However, contrary to expectation, it was the high and medium sensation seeking current smokers who estimated the greater risk and the lows who guessed the lowest risk! If we are to believe these data, about two thirds of the high and medium sensation seekers, in contrast to one third of the low sensation seekers, believe that there is a 50% chance of a heavy smoker developing lung cancer! How could anyone continue to smoke if they really thought the odds for disaster were that high? The answer may be that few of these smokers regard themselves as "heavy smokers" and according to their reports most are not; only 11% smoked one or more packs a day. Almost all of them are smoking brands advertised as "light" (on tars and nicotine). In retrospect, it would have been better to ask about the chances of developing lung cancer for anyone who smoked at all.

It is interesting that high and medium sensation seekers estimate this risk as higher than do lows in contradiction to their general tendency to minimize risk relative to lows. It may be more important for those lows who are smokers to deny the risk in what they are doing than it is for the highs. The relationship was not found among those lows who quit smoking, indicating that low sensation seekers judge the risk as higher when they have given up the risky activity: 64% of the lows who quit smoking saw the activity as leading to cancer in half of the heavy smokers, but only 35% of the lows who were still smoking estimated this kind of high risk. In contrast, an equal percentage of high sensation seekers (60%) estimated the maximal risk regardless of whether they were currently smoking or not.

These data are consistent with sensation seekers expectations of positive (sensation seeking) or negative (anxiety) affect in responses to hypothetical situations equated for risk appraisal (Zuckerman, 1979b). In response to situations that both high and low sensation seekers regard as equally risky, like taking a dangerous trip or taking an unknown drug in an experiment, the highs anticipate experiencing more positive affect than anxiety, while the lows anticipate more anxiety than positive feelings. The attitude of the high sensation seeker seems to be: "Yes, it's risky but I know everything will turn out fine for me and I will feel good." The attitude of the low sensation seeker is: "Everything bad that can happen will happen, and I will be devastated."

Situational Determinants of Smoking and Sensation Seeking

Although more high sensation seekers smoke than lows, some lows do smoke but perhaps for different reasons. As the active drug in smoking is nicotine, a central nervous system stimulant, the most obvious motive for smoking is to maintain or increase arousal. However, some smokers smoke more when they are emotionally aroused, with the idea that smoking calms them. This effect may be due simply to conditioned relief, distraction, or similar factors, or it could actually be due to individual differences in physiological reactions to nicotine.

One approach to exploring the motivation of smokers has been the development of situational smoking questionnaires (Frith, 1971; O'Connor, 1980, 1985) which list different types of situations and ask respondents to indicate the likelihood of their smoking in each situation. Frith (1971) factor analyzed his scale and found two primary factors: a generalization of smoking or the readiness to smoke in almost all situations, and a bipolar arousal factor. At one pole of the latter factor are smokers who tend to smoke primarily in high arousal situations, usually emotionally charged ones; at the other pole are smokers who are more likely to smoke in low arousal situations of relaxation or monotony. O'Connor (1980, 1985) found two similar first factors, generalized smoking and arousal-nonarousal, although he calls the latter factor "stressful-nonstressful." But in addition to these two factors, O'Connor reported a factor reflecting attention-demands, and one depending on the solitary versus social nature of the situations.

Both Frith and O'Connor found that females tended to smoke more in situations of high emotional stress than males, and persons of both sexes scoring high on neuroticism also tended to smoke more than stable persons in stressful situations. Introverts, in contrast to extraverts, were more likely to smoke during tasks requiring high attention, while extraverts were more likely to smoke in non-attention demanding situations including socializing ones.

In order to study the motivations for smoking that might be related to sensation seeking, we decided to develop a new smoking questionnaire. Many new items were added to some of those used by Frith and O'Connor in order to provide more markers for the factors suggested by their analyses. A total of 62 situational smoking items were included in the questionnaire. The questionnaire was given to 420 undergraduate students. Of these only 141 were current or past smokers and therefore could fill out the questionnaire in regard to their smoking habits.

The responses to the 62 situational items plus one item which asked how much they smoke were factor analyzed using principal components. The first three factors accounted for 64.6% of the total variance and additional factors beyond these showed only very gradual changes in Eigenvalues, so on the basis of the visual Scree test it was decided to rotate only these three factors. A varimax rotation appeared to provide the best definitions of the factors. The resultant factors with illustrative items from the highest loading ones are listed below.

Factor 1 was called *Relaxation or Boredom (RB)* and indicates the desire to smoke in low arousal situations whether positive (relaxation) or negative (boredom). High loading items include: while listening to music; having a restful evening alone; while watching television; while sitting around with nothing to do; waiting for a bus, train, or airplane with nothing to do; while riding in an automobile; immediately after a meal; when in a very boring situation.

Factor 2 was labeled *Attention-Concentration (AC)* and indicates the need to smoke in order to maintain arousal in situations requiring focused attention. High loading items include: while doing a job requiring total concentration; filling in a complicated form; when immersed in an interesting hobby; when trying to help someone who is emotionally upset; when searching through a long list of names; while playing a game; while giving a talk.

Factor 3 was described as *Negative Emotional Arousal (NegEm)* and reflects the paradoxical use of smoking to reduce unpleasant arousal. Sample items are: when you are emotionally upset; after hearing that a friend has been involved in an accident; when you are angry; after hearing some bad news; when you are anxious; while being criticized; waiting to hear an important result; at a party where you don't know anyone.

On the basis of these factor analytic results, items were assigned to the factor on which they had the highest loadings, and scales were devised for each of the three smoking factors.

The SSSV and the Smoking Questionnaire (SQ) were given to 651 subjects

Table 4.6. Gender and Sensation Seeking as Sources of Variance in Scores from a Smoking Questionnaire

SS	Gender	A–C	Means on Situation Scales*	
			R–B	NegEm
Low	Males	17.4	26.2	14.6
	Females	20.9	40.8	24.1
Medium	Males	17.5	29.5	16.8
	Females	18.8	34.4	22.7
High	Males	22.6	41.1	23.8
	Females	22.7	43.6	27.7

F Ratios ANOVA

Gender (df = 1/162)	.70	4.78†	7.28‡
SS (df = 2/162)	3.08†	5.94‡	4.59‡
Gender X SS (df = 2/162)	.23	1.01	.45

F Ratios ANCOVA

Gender (df = 1/161)	.33	5.40†	8.50‡
SS (df = 2/161)	1.55	4.48†	3.10†
Gender X SS (df = 2/161)	.13	1.14	.34

*A–C = attention concentration; R–B = relaxation or boredom; NegEm = negative emotional arousal.
†$p < .05$
‡$p < .01$

from a new sample of students. Of these, 202 or 31% were either past or present smokers. However, complete records were only obtained from 172 of these subjects and these were used in further analyses. The original distribution of SSS Total scores was used to divide the subjects into groups of low, medium, and high sensation seekers. As there was a relationship between sensation seeking and smoking in the original group, there were more high sensation seekers in this smoker sample who filled out the situational smoking part of the questionnaire. Table 4.6 shows the means of low, medium, and high sensation seekers, divided by gender, on the three situation smoking scales derived from the factor analysis of the previous sample. The three situation smoking factor scales correlated quite highly among themselves and all three scales correlated with the self-rating of how many cigarettes were smoked daily (rs .61 to .65). A Multiple Analysis of Covariance (MANCOVA) was done with gender of subjects (male versus female), sensation seeking (low, middle, high) and their interaction as the main sources of variance, the three situation factor scores (A-C, R-B, and NegEm) as the dependent variables, and the extent of smoking as the covariate. The univariate results for the ANOVA and ANCOVA analyses are also presented in Table 4.6.

The ANCOVA effects of sex were significant for both the Relaxation-Boredom and the Negative Emotional Arousal scales, but not for the Attention-Concentration scale. Females scored higher than males on both of the former scales. Sensation seeking was also a significant source of variance for the Relaxation-Boredom and Negative Emotional Arousal Scales with high sensation seekers showing higher scores than both middle and low groups. The effect of sensation seeking on the Attention-Concentration scale had been significant before application of covariance for control of the extent of smoking, but in the covariance analysis the effect was attenuated. None of the interactions between gender and sensation seeking even approached significance.

The sex difference on the Negative Emotional Arousal scale is similar to the results of Frith (1971) and O'Connor (1980) who also found that females report smoking more in emotionally stressful situations. However, the finding in the current study that females report smoking more in relaxing or boring situations was not expected. It may have something to do with the change in the sex ratio of smokers in our college population. Because smoking may be facilitated by social influence, the greater presence of smokers in the female dormitories or other places of congregation during hours of relaxation may increase female smoking in these situations.

Sensation seeking was only expected to be related to the Relaxation-Boredom situational influence where people presumably smoke to increase arousal. Sensation seekers are more susceptible to boredom and feel best in states of relatively high arousal, thus they would be expected to smoke in conditions where stimulation is minimal and the environment is monotonous. The results support this hypothesis. However, sensation seekers were also high on the Negative Emotional Arousal factor even though this effect was not quite as strong as the one for Relaxation-Boredom. Sensation seekers, therefore, seem to smoke in conditions where the desire would be to increase arousal and also in situations where the inclination for most would be to reduce negatively toned arousal. Perhaps, high sensation seekers do not share the need of others to reduce arousal in negatively toned situations, but instead attempt to maintain arousal in order to cope with the situation. Hearing that a friend has been involved in an accident, building up courage to do something, expressing a point of view to someone who does not agree, at a party where one does not know anyone, are all examples of situations where the high level of emotional arousal may facilitate adaptive behavior. If the optimal level of arousal of the high sensation seeker is higher than that of the low, then the same high level of arousal that is disruptive of adaptive behavior for the low may be facilitative for the high sensation seeker.

However, there is a more parsimonious hypothesis concerning the method used to measure the two situational factors. Even after partialling out the influence of the item referring to smoking frequency, the two scales correlated

.80. We will have to develop purer scales or use scoring methods that eliminate the correlation between scales in order to distinguish between the situational factors. With added discriminant power such scales might show that the relationship of sensation seeking to smoking is more strictly explainable by the desire to increase arousal in low stimulation situations through the stimulation of nicotine.

We are currently conducting an experiment in which high and low sensation seekers are put in a social isolation situation, some with cigarettes and others without cigarettes to smoke. Our prediction is that the high sensation seekers will show more disturbance in response to boredom as a function of whether or not they are allowed to smoke. Additional experiments are planned for types of stress more likely to produce high states of negative emotional arousal.

Reflections on Personality and Health

As the emphasis in medicine shifts toward prevention, there is an increasing need to consider the role of individual differences in the etiology of physical illness. There is one role of personality in which the illness is an incidental result of the biological make-up of a particular personality type. The low sensation seeker may be more biologically prone to hypertension, despite the fact that the high sensation seeker has more habits that should elevate blood pressure, either directly as in the case of alcohol, or indirectly as when engaging in risky activities. The vulnerability of low sensation seekers may be due to an overactive or oversensitive noradrenergic system that makes them prone to overreact through cardiovascular mechanisms.

Apart from medications that act directly on the noradrenergic mechanism, a stress reduction program is entirely appropriate for such individuals. However, such a program may have to be tailored somewhat differently for the occasional high sensation seeker who develops the disorder. Trying to reduce his or her normal sensation seeking behavior may create more stress and higher risk for cardiovascular disease than letting them resume many of their normal activities after the blood pressure is brought under some degree of control. The medications that are used to control blood pressure may affect high and low sensation seekers quite differently leading to a problem of non-compliance in the highs. Systematic collection of data on catecholamines and their enzymes in patients should be part of the diagnostic process. There is no point in using a drug whose function is to reduce the activity in some neurotransmitter system if activity is normal or subnormal in that system. Collection of personality data along with biochemical analyses in research studies could elucidate the role of individual differences in physical illness.

Another role of personality in physical illness is mediated more directly through the actual behaviors associated with the personality type. The role of smoking, drug and alcohol abuse, and dietary habits in various diseases is recognized, although there is some debate about the inferences to be drawn from these correlational data. Only the outcome of many large-scale longitudinal studies can test the efficacy of preventative medicine. In the meantime, individuals must assess their tolerance for risk against the losses in reward of giving up certain appetites or activities.

There really is such a beast as the "addictive personality." The typical weight gain after giving up smoking is well-documented. I recently observed an individual who gained 50 pounds shortly after giving up smoking. Interestingly, as a child he was hyperactive and highly intelligent. His current activity is largely restricted to a business involving artistic interests, but involving a great deal of stress. In giving up smoking he has exchanged one type of risk for another. There is such a thing as a generalized appetite for sensation that is involved in eating as well as smoking. At a therapeutic community where I once consulted, I observed drug-deprived addicts smoke and drink coffee, the only two drugs allowed, with an avidity that was unbelievable. Among those who became paraprofessionals and were allowed to drink, many former heroin addicts were well on their way to alcoholism. Certain kinds of impulsive behaviors, regarded by the community as antisocial, were also a problem for graduates of the program. Recognition of the role of individual differences is essential to anticipation of problems in therapy and the design of effective remedial programs.

There is a current emphasis upon cognitive modes of therapy and explanations for many disorders. The limitations of simple cognitive methods are illustrated in some of our data. Most of the smokers, with the exception of the low sensation seekers, not only seemed cognizant of the risk involved in smoking but actually exaggerated it. No matter how explict they make the message and no matter how large they make the printing on the side of the cigarette package, most smokers will not be dissuaded by the emphasis on risk. Most drug abusers are high sensation seekers and most of them know of friends who have died or gone to jail as a consequence of their drug use. The riskiness of the drug life actually enhances it for some of the higher sensation seekers.

If cognitive approaches are used they must be more subtle and aimed at the basic values and motivations of the user. Donohew, Helm, Cook, and Shatzer (1986) have recently completed a study on the effects of exposure to prevention messages on marijuana use. At various points in the presentation, subjects indicated whether they wanted further exposure or would prefer to stop. They found a curious interaction between sensation seeking trait and usage of marijuana in regard to exposure preferences. Subjects showing the greatest preference for exposure to the message were high sensation seekers who *did not* use marijuana and low sensation seekers who *did* use the drug. The relevance of the message seems to determine its interest. Young high sensation seekers (high school students in this case) who do not currently use marijuana are a group who are tempted, whereas those who are already using it have either discounted or come to terms with the risks involved. The message is of little interest to low sensation seekers who do not use marijuana for they have already accepted the message. However lows who do use the drug are more concerned about the risks and avid for information than the highs who use it. These interesting results show how a knowledge of personality differences may be crucial in even getting persons to expose themselves to messages. In this regard, it is interesting that the U.S. government is going to require cigarette companies to vary the content of the risk message on the side of the cigarette pack. Someone seems to know that habituation may occur rapidly with repetition of an unwelcome message.

References

Alexander, F. (1939). Emotional factors in essential hypertension: Presentation of a tentative hypothesis. *Psychosomatic Medicine, 1*, 173–179.

Ballenger, J.C., Post, R.M., Jimerson, D.C., Lake, C.R., Murphy, D.L., Zuckerman, M., & Cronin, C. (1983). Biochemical correlates of personality traits in normals: An exploratory study. *Personality and Individual Differences, 4*, 615–625.

Carrol, E.N., Zuckerman, M., & Vogel, W.H. (1982). A test of the optimal level of arousal theory of sensation seeking. *Journal of Personality and Social Psychology, 42*, 572–575.

Charney, D.S., & Heninger, G.R. (1986). Abnormal regulation of noradrenergic function in panic disorders. *Archives of General Psychiatry, 11*, 1042–1054.

Donohew, L., Helm, D., Cook, P., & Shatzer, M.J. (1986). Sensation seeking, marijuana use, and responses to prevention messages: Implications for public health campaigns. Unpublished manuscript.

Frith, C.D. (1971). Smoking behaviour and its relation to the smokers immediate experience. *British Journal of Social and Clinical Psychology, 10*, 73–78.

von Knorring, L., Oreland, L., & Winblad, B. (1984). Personality traits related to monoamine oxidase activity in platelets. *Psychiatry Research, 12*, 11–26.

Kulcsár, S., Kutor, L., & Arató, M. (1984). Sensation seeking and its biological correlates, and its relation to vestibulo-ocular functions. In H. Bonarius, G. van Heck, & N. Smid (Eds.), *Personality psychology in Europe: Theoretical & empirical developments* (pp. 327–346). Lisse, The Netherlands: Swets & Zeitinger.

Litle, P.A. (1986). Effects of a stressful movie and music on mood and physiological arousal in relation to sensation seeking. Doctoral dissertation, University of Delaware, Newark.

O'Connor, K. (1980). Individual differences in situational preference amongst smokers. *Personality and Individual Differences, 1*, 249–257.

O'Connor, K. (1985). A model of situational preference amongst smokers. *Personality and Individual Differences, 6*, 151–160.

Potter, W.Z., Muscettola, G., & Goodwin, F.K. (1983). Sources of variance in clinical studies of MHPG. In J.W. Maas (Ed.), *MHPG: Basic mechanisms and psychopathology* (pp. 145–165). New York: Academic Press.

Schalling, D., & Svensson, J. (1984). Blood pressure and personality. *Personality and Individual Differences, 5*, 41–51.

Umberkoman-Wiita, B., Vogel, W.H., & Wiita, P.J. (1981). Some biochemical and behavioral (sensation seeking)correlates in healthy adults. *Research Communications in Psychology, Psychiatry and Behavior, 6*, 330–316.

Zuckerman, M. (1979a). *Sensation seeking: Beyond the optimal level of arousal*. Hillsdale, NJ: Lawrence Erlbaum Associates.

Zuckerman, M. (1979b). Sensation seeking and risk taking. In C.E. Izard (Ed.), *Emotions in personality and psychopathology* (pp. 163–197). New York: Plenum Press.

Zuckerman, M. (1984). Sensation seeking: A comparative approach to a human trait. *Behavioral and Brain Sciences*, 7, 413–471.

Zuckerman, M., & Neeb, M. (1980). Demographic influences in sensation seeking and expressions of sensation seeking in religion, smoking, and driving habits. *Personality and Individual Differences*, 1, 197–206.

5

The Experience, Expression, and Control of Anger

Charles D. Spielberger, Susan S. Krasner,
and Eldra P. Solomon

In this chapter, Spielberger, Krasner, and Solomon concentrate upon the sensation that is called anger, hostility, or aggression. They liken anger to a state emotion and hostility to a trait, whereas the label aggression is reserved for the behavioral expression of the first two. They refer to the structure of these three concepts as the *AHA! Syndrome*. The chapter begins with a thorough review of the history of the relationship between anger and psychosomatics. Also featured is a discussion of the role of anger in the Type A behavior pattern and on the nature of anger itself. Following a brief review of the history of attempts to measure hostility and anger, we are introduced to the State-Trait Anger Scale (STAS) developed by Spielberger and his colleagues. The authors then provide an in-depth review of research and thinking on the nature of the expression of anger; that is, whether it is directed inward (suppressed) or outward (expressed). The nature and meaning of the control of anger is also reviewed. We are presented with the principal psychometric data related to the development of the Anger EXpression Scale (AX), which measures anger-in, anger-out, and anger-control. In concluding, the authors explain the need for scales such as the STAS and AX and describe their usefulness in individual difference and health research.

—Editor

Anger, hostility, and aggression have long been regarded as important factors in essential hypertension and coronary heart disease (see Diamond, 1982). Almost 50 years ago, Franz Alexander (1939) theorized that the strenuous efforts of hypertensives to suppress their angry feelings resulted in chronic activation of the cardiovascular system, and, eventually, to fixed elevations in blood pressure. Impressive evidence of a strong relationship between suppressed hostility ("anger-in") and hypertension has also been reported by Harburg and his associates (Esler et al., 1977; Gentry, Chesney,

Gary, Hall, & Harburg, 1982; Harburg, Erfurt, Chape, Schull, & Schork, 1973; Harburg, Blakelock, & Roeper, 1979).

Flanders Dunbar (1943), a pioneer in psychosomatic medicine, was among the first to note an association between aggression and coronary heart disease (CHD). She identified a "coronary personality" in CHD patients, whom she described as ambitious, hard-driving, and markedly aggressive, with a strong need for achievement and success. Friedman and Rosenman (1959, 1974) observed similar attitudes and behaviors in CHD patients, which they labeled the Type A Behavior Pattern (TABP). The TABP is an action-emotion syndrome characterized by competitiveness, agressiveness, achievement striving, impatience, and an extreme sense of time urgency. According to Friedman and Rosenman: "Persons possessing this pattern are quite prone to exhibit a free floating but extraordinarily well-rationalized hostility, which was likely to flare up under very diverse conditions" (1974, p. 59).

Evidence of a strong association between the TABP and CHD was reported by Matthews, Glass, Rosenman, and Bortner (1977). In a prospective study of Type-A and Type-B persons, they also found that individuals who developed CHD were rated significantly higher than age-matched healthy controls on each of the following characteristics: "Potential for hostility;" "Anger directed outward;" "Subject gets angry more than once a week;" "Irritation at waiting in lines;" "Subject's answers are vigorous;" "Explosive voice modulation;" and "Competitive in games with peers." All seven characteristics are either directly related to anger/hostility or possibly motivated by anger. Thus, the experience and expression of anger and hostility would seem to be a major coronary-prone component of the TABP.

The Type A characteristic style of coping may also influence how they express anger. Typically, Type As readily admit to having a fiery temper or insist that they never get angry (Jenkins, Zyzanski, & Rosenman, 1978). Noting these conflicting tendencies, Jenkins and co-workers (1978) concluded that the Type A deals with angry feelings either by undercontrol and frequent expression, or overcontrol and unrealistic denial.

The results of recent studies of the association of hostility with coronary artery disease (CAD) provide further evidence of a significant relationship between anger/hostility and CHD. Williams, Barefoot, and Shekelle (1985) found that hostility and cynicism were related to the presence and severity of CAD, as measured by coronary angiography. Similarly, Dembroski, Mac-Dougall, Williams, and Haney (1984) reported that potential for hostility was associated with CAD, but only for patients who suppressed their anger (anger-in). These findings highlight the importance of assessing the suppression and control of anger/hostility, in addition to measuring how often angry feelings are experienced and expressed.

Although evidence is mounting of an association of anger, hostility, and aggression with CHD, there remains considerable ambiguity and inconsistency with regard to how these constructs are defined and even less agreement on how they should be measured. In this chapter we will endeavor to clarify the nature of anger, hostility, and aggression as psychological constructs. Conceptual distinctions and empirical research on anger as an emotional state, and individual differences in the experience and expression of anger as personality traits, will also be briefly reviewed. The construction and validation of the *Anger EXpression* (AX) Scale, a psychometric inventory for assessing the experience, expression, and control of anger, will then be described in some detail.

Anger, Hostility, and Aggression: The AHA! Syndrome

In the psychological and psychiatric literature, anger, hostility, and aggression generally refer to different though related phenomena, but these terms are often used interchangeably (Berkowitz, 1962; Buss, 1961). Given substantial overlap in the prevailing conceptual definitions of anger, hostility, and aggression, and the variety of operational procedures used to assess these constructs, we have referred to them, collectively, as the AHA! Syndrome (Spielberger et al., 1985). Progress in research on the role of anger, hostility, and aggression in the etiology of essential hypertension and CHD requires conceptual clarification of the components of the AHA! Syndrome, and the construction of objective, reliable, and valid measures of each component.

On the basis of a careful examination of the research literature on anger, hostility, and aggression, Spielberger, Jacobs, Russell, and Crane (1983) proposed the following as working definitions of these constructs:

> The concept of anger usually refers to an emotional state that consists of feelings that vary in intensity, from mild irritation or annoyance to intense fury and rage. Although hostility usually involves angry feelings, this concept has the connotation of a complex set of attitudes that motivate aggressive behaviors directed toward destroying objects or injuring other people. . . . While anger and hostility refer to feelings and attitudes, the concept of aggression generally implies destructive or punitive behavior directed towards other persons or objects (p. 16).

The emotion of anger is clearly at the core of the AHA! Syndrome, but different aspects of this emotion are typically emphasized in various definitions. For example, Buss (1961) includes facial-skeletal and autonomic components in his definition of anger reactions, and Feshbach (1964) conceptualizes anger as an undifferentiated state of emotional arousal. Schachter (1971) and Novaco (1975) include both physiological and cognitive factors in their definitions of anger as an emotional state. Such ambiguities and inconsistencies in definitions of the nature of anger as a psychological construct are reflected in the procedures that have been developed to assess anger.

The earliest efforts to assess anger and hostility were based on clinical interviews, behavioral observations, and projective techniques such as the Rorschach inkblots and the Thematic Apperception Test. Beginning in the

1950s, a number of self-report psychometric scales were developed to measure hostility (e.g., Buss & Durkee, 1957; Caine, Foulds, & Hope, 1967; Cook & Medley, 1954; Schultz, 1954; Siegel, 1956), but the phenomenological experience of anger as an emotional state, that is, angry feelings, was largely neglected in psychological theory and research.

The need to distinguish between anger and hostility was explicitly recognized in the early 1970s by the appearance of three anger scales in the psychological literature: The Reaction Inventory (RI), the Anger Inventory (AI), and the Anger Self-Report (ASR). The RI was developed by Evans and Stangeland (1971) to assess the degree to which anger was evoked in a number of specific situations (e.g., "People pushing into line"). Subjects report the amount of anger they believe they would experience in each situation by rating themselves on a 5-point scale, from "Not at all" to "Very much." Novaco's (1975) Anger Inventory is similar in conception and format to the RI, consisting of 90 statements that describe anger-provoking incidents ("Being called a liar," "Someone spits at you"). Subjects rate, on a 5-point scale, the degree to which each incident would anger or provoke them.

The ASR was designed by Zelin, Adler, and Myerson (1972) to assess "awareness of anger" and different modes of anger expression. In validating this scale, they found that the ASR scores of psychiatric patients correlated significantly with psychiatrists' ratings of anger, and that college students' ASR "awareness of anger" scores correlated significantly with acquaintances' peer ratings of angry feelings. Because the ASR and the RI have been used in only one or two studies over the past 15 years, the construct validity of these scales has yet to be firmly established. While the AI has been used more often in research than the other anger measures, Biaggio, Supplee, and Curtis (1981) found no significant correlations of this scale with self and observer ratings of anger and hostility. Moreover, over a brief 2-week interval, the test-retest stability of the AI was only .17.

Empirical efforts to assess anger, as distinguished from hostility and aggression, reflect an important theoretical development in research on the AHA! Syndrome. There are, however, a number of limitations inherent in the three anger scales described above. For example, none of these scales adequately distinguishes between anger as an emotional state (angry feelings) and individual differences in anger-proneness as a personality trait. Moreover, in inquiring about hypothetical anger reactions to provocative situations, the RI and the AI confound the experience and expression of anger with situational determinants of anger reactions.

In order to measure the fundamental properties of anger, it is essential to assess the intensity of angry feelings that are experienced at a particular time, the frequency that anger is experienced, and whether anger is held in (suppressed) or expressed in aggressive behavior directed toward other persons or objects in the environment. Recent research further suggests that it is also important to evaluate the degree to which a person endeavors to control anger (Spielberger et al., 1985).

The State-Trait Anger Scale (STAS), which is analogous in conception and similar in format to the State-Trait Anxiety Inventory (Spielberger, 1983; Spielberger, Gorsuch, & Lushene, 1970), was designed to assess the intensity of anger as an emotional state and individual differences in anger proneness as a personality trait (Spielberger, 1980; Spielberger et al., 1983). State anger (S-Anger) was defined as an emotional state or condition that consists of subjective feelings of irritation, annoyance, fury, and rage, with concommitant activation or arousal of the autonomic nervous system. It was further assumed that S-Anger will vary in *intensity* and fluctuate over time as a function of perceived affronts, being attacked or treated unfairly, or frustration resulting from the blocking of goal-directed behavior. In constructing the STAS, Trait anger (T-Anger) was operationally defined in terms of individual differences in the *frequency* that S-Anger was experienced over time. It was assumed that persons high in T-Anger would be more likely to perceive a wider range of situations as anger-provoking (e.g., annoying, irritating, frustrating) than individuals low in T-Anger, and to respond to such situations with elevations in S-Anger. In addition to experiencing S-Anger more often, persons high in T-Anger tend to experience more intense elevations in S-Anger whenever annoying or frustrating conditions are encountered.

Examples of items in the STAS S-Anger scale are: "I am furious;" "I feel angry;" "I feel irritated;" "I am burned up." In responding to each item, subjects report the intensity of their angry feelings, "right now," by rating themselves on the following 4-point scale: "Not at all;" "Somewhat;" "Moderately so;" "Very much so." Examples of items in the STAS T-Anger scale are: "I have a fiery temper;" "I am a hotheaded person;" "It makes me furious when I am criticized in front of others." In responding to these items, subjects indicate how they generally feel by rating themselves on the following 4-point scale: "Almost never;" "Sometimes;" "Often;" "Almost always."

The critical importance of measuring the characteristic ways in which people express or suppress their anger has become increasingly apparent in research on the assessment of state and trait anger. The expression of anger must be distinguished, conceptually and empirically, from the experience of anger as an emotional state and individual differences in anger-proneness as a personality trait. Research on anger expression is briefly reviewed below.

The Expression of Anger

In previous research on anger expression, individuals were typically classified as "anger-out" if they expressed anger toward other persons or objects in the environment (e.g., Funkenstein, King, & Drolette, 1954). "Anger-out" generally involves an increase in S-Anger and the manifestation of aggressive behavior. Anger directed outward may be expressed in physical acts such as assaulting other persons, destroying objects, and slamming doors, or expressed in criticism, insults, verbal threats, and the extreme use of profanity.

Both physical and verbal manifestations of anger may be expressed directly toward the source of provocation or frustration, or indirectly toward persons or objects closely associated with, or symbolic of the provoking agent.

Persons who direct their anger inward toward the ego or self, or who hold in (suppress) their anger, are classified as "anger-in" (Averill, 1982; Funkenstein et al., 1954; Tavris, 1982). The psychoanalytic conception of anger turned inward, directed toward the ego or self, implies that feelings of guilt and depression, rather than anger, will be experienced (Alexander & French, 1948). With this type of anger-in, thoughts and memories relating to the anger provoking situation, and even the feelings of anger themselves, may be repressed or denied. In contrast, suppressed anger is consciously experienced as an emotional state, S-Anger, which may vary in intensity and fluctuate over time as a function of the provoking circumstances.

The conceptual distinction between anger-in and anger-out was used by Funkenstein and co-workers (1954) in their classic studies of the effects of anger expression on the cardiovascular system. Pulse rate and blood pressure were measured in healthy college students exposed to anger-inducing laboratory conditions. In addition to closely observing the students' behavior, post-stress interviews were conducted to determine what emotions were actually experienced. Students who became angry during the experiment and directed their anger at the investigator or the laboratory situation, were classified as anger-out; those who suppressed their anger and/or directed it at themselves were classified as anger-in. The increase in pulse rate for the anger in group was three times greater than for the anger out group. Significant differences between the two groups were also found for three other ballistocardiograph measures.

In a major research program on hypertension, Harburg and his associates investigated relationships between anger expression, elevated blood pressure (BP), and hypertension (Harburg et al., 1979; Harburg et al., 1973; Harburg & Hauenstein, 1980; Harburg, Schull, Erfurt, & Schork, 1970). Anger-in and anger-out were operationally defined on the basis of responses to a self-report questionnaire that described several hypothetical anger-provoking situations, such as being verbally abused by a police officer or a landlord. Persons who reported they would get angry or mad, and show it, were classified as anger out. Those who reported they would either not get angry, or that they would become angry but keep it in, were classified as anger-in. Individuals residing in high stress areas who used anger-in coping styles, which Harburg labeled "suppressed hostility," had significantly higher BP than those who "expressed hostility."

Gentry (1972) and his colleagues (Gentry, Chesney, Hall, & Harburg, 1981; Gentry et al., 1982) have reported findings based on intensive analyses of Harburg and co-workers' (1973) data that help to clarify the relationships between habitual anger coping styles, elevated BP, and the risk of hypertension. Subjects were classified as low, medium, or high in anger expression on the basis of the proportion of their anger-out responses to each of five different hypothetical, anger-provoking interpersonal situations. High anger-out subjects had significantly lower diastolic BP and slightly lower systolic BP than individuals classified as medium or low in expressed anger.

The findings by Harburg, Gentry, and their colleagues of an association between anger expression, elevated BP, and hypertension clearly demonstrate that anger-in and anger-out have different effects on the cardiovascular system. There are, however, a number of problems in the procedures they employed in assessing anger expression that make it difficult to interpret and generalize their results. For example, Harburg's questionnaire was designed to assess anger expression in adults residing in a large city, which may not be appropriate for other populations. He also classified his subjects into anger-in and anger-out groups on the basis of their responses to only two hypothetical situations, which many of them had never actually experienced. Moreover, Gentry used Harburg's questionnaire in classifying his subjects into low, medium, and high "anger out" groups, so the ecological validity of his stressor situations is also questionable. The problem of ecological validity can be resolved by assessing individual differences in how often people generally experience anger (T-Anger), engage in aggressive behaviors when they feel angry or furious (anger-out), or suppress their angry feelings (anger-in).

The fact that Harburg and Gentry classified persons as anger in who reported they did not feel angry in a particular anger-provoking situation raises important conceptual issues. This procedure equates individuals who do not experience anger with those who experience and suppress their angry feelings. Rosenzweig (1976, 1978) attributes very different personality dynamics to "impunitive" persons who do not experience anger in anger-provoking situations, and "intrapunitive" persons who turn anger in, often blaming themselves for provoking anger in others. The problem of differentiating between the experience and the expression of anger can be resolved by measuring the intensity of the experience of S-Anger, and the frequency that S-Anger is expressed in behavior (anger-out) or suppressed (anger-in). Efforts to construct a self-report rating scale to assess individual differences in anger expression are described in the following section.

Assessment of Anger Expression

Because anger expression was implicitly defined by Funkenstein, Harburg, and Gentry as a unidimensional construct, it was assumed that this construct could be most meaningfully assessed by a single, bipolar rating scale. As a first step in constructing the *Anger EXpression* (AX) Scale, working definitions of anger-in and anger-out were formulated. Anger-in was defined on the basis of how often an individual experiences but does *not* express angry feelings, rather than in terms of the psychoanalytic construct of anger turned aganist the ego. Anger-out was defined in terms of the frequency that an individual engages in aggressive behavior when motivated by angry feelings. Consistent with these definitions, items were written with content ranging from strong inhibition or suppression of angry feelings (anger-in) to the extreme expression of anger toward other persons or objects in the environment (anger-out). Examples of AX Scale anger-in and anger-out items are:

1. "I boil inside, but I don't show it."
2. "I keep things in."
3. "I say nasty things."
4. "I lose my temper."

In contrast to the procedures used by Funkenstein and Harburg of assigning subjects to dichotomous anger-in and anger-out categories, the AX Scale was designed to measure a continuum of individual differences in how often anger was held in or expressed. The same rating-scale format used to assess T-Anger in the *State-Trait Anger Scale* (Spielberger, 1980) was adapted for the AX Scale, but the instructions differed markedly from those previously used with other trait measures. Rather than asking subjects to respond to each item according to how they generally feel, they are instructed to report ". . . how *often* you *generally* react or *behave* in the manner described (when you) feel *angry* or *furious*" by rating themselves on the following 4-point scale: (1) Almost never; (2) Sometimes; (3) Often; (4) Almost always.

In a study of the relationship between anger expression and blood pressure, Johnson (1984) administered a 30-item preliminary version of the AX Scale to 1,114 high school students. To verify that the AX items measured a unitary psychological construct, students' responses to the individual items were factored separately for males and females. Although we originally intended to develop a continuous, unidimensional bipolar measure of anger expression, the results of the factor analyses suggested that the AX items were tapping two independent, underlying dimensions. On the basis of the content of the items loading these factors, they were labeled Anger/In and Anger/Out. Most items had strong loadings on one of these factors and negligible loadings on the other.

Given the clarity and strength of the Anger/In and Anger/Out factors, the striking similarity (invariance) of these factors for males and females, and the large samples on which these analyses were based, we modified our test construction strategy to develop separate subscales for measuring anger-in and anger-out. The selection of the final set of 20 items for the AX Scale, and for subscales to measure anger-in and anger-out, was based on further factor analyses of the AX items and on subscale item-remainder correlations for the items comprising these scales (Spielberger et al., 1985).

Eight items with high loadings for both sexes on the Anger/In factor, ranging from .58 to .72 (mdn = .67), and negligible loadings on AX/Out (mdn = −.04), were selected for the AX/In subscale. In a similar manner, eight items with high loadings on AX/Out (mdn = .59) and negligible loadings on AX/In (mdn = −.01) were selected for the AX/Out subscale. The internal consistency of the AX/In and AX/Out subscales, as measured by alpha coefficients, ranged from .73 to .84, which was reasonably satisfactory for brief 8-item scales. The item-remainder correlations for the AX/In items were surprisingly large (mdn = .53); those for the AX/Out subscale, though somewhat smaller, were also quite satisfactory (mdn = .44). Eigenvalues and factor loadings for the AX Scale, and item-remainder correlations and alpha coefficients for the AX/In and AX/Out subscales, are reported in Table 5.1.

Johnson (1984) and Pollans (1983) found essentially zero correlations between the AX/In and AX/Out subscales for both males and females in large samples of high school and college students; similar findings have also been obtained for other populations (Spielberger, in press). Thus, the Anger/In and Anger/Out subscales are empirically independent, as well as factorially orthogonal. Clearly, the Anger/In and Anger/Out subscales assess two independent anger-expression dimensions.

Several items that were intended to measure the middle region of the anger-in/anger-out continuum were included in the original AX Scale item pool. Three of these items ("Control my temper;" "Keep my cool;" "Calm down faster") were retained for the final version of the 20-item AX Scale because they had substantial loadings on both the Anger/In and Anger/Out factors. These items appear to measure anger control, which logically cuts across both modes of anger expression.

Pollans (1983) found evidence of an AX Scale "anger control" factor for college males, but not for females for whom the anger control items had negative loadings on the Anger/Out factor. The emergence of anger control as an aspect of anger expression stimulated the development of an AX anger control (AX/Con) subscale. After considering research findings in several studies in which the 20-item AX Scale was used to assess anger-in and anger-out, the construction of an 8-item AX/Con subscale is described.

Research with the Anger EXpression (AX) Scale

Johnson (1984) administered the AX Scale and the *State-Trait Personality Inventory* (STPI: Spielberger, 1979) to a sample of 1,114 high school students for whom he also obtained resting measures of systolic (SBP) and diastolic (DBP) blood pressure. The STPI is comprised of six 10-item subscales, which measure state and trait anger, anxiety, and curiosity. Significant positive correlations were found between the AX/Out and AX/In subscales and the STPI T-Anger scale for both males and females. These findings suggested that individuals who more often experience anger are more likely to both express and suppress their anger than persons who experience anger less frequently. The fact that the correlations were substantially larger for AX/Out than for AX/In further suggested that individuals who experience anger more frequently are more likely to express anger toward other persons or objects in the environment than to suppress it.

Johnson also found highly significant positive correlations of AX/In scores with both SBP and DBP, and small but significant negative correlations of AX/Out with SBP for both males and females. Thus, holding anger in was associated with higher blood pressure, especially higher SBP, whereas per-

Table 5.1. Factor Loadings, Item-Remainder Correlations, and Alpha Coefficients for the AX Anger/In and Anger/Out Subscales for High School Students

Item Content	Factor Loadings				Item Correlations*			
	Anger/In		Anger/Out		AX/In		AX/Out	
	M	F	M	F	M	F	M	F
Withdraw from people	.72	.68	−.05	−.04	.63	.57		
Pout or sulk	.72	.65	−.04	−.10	.63	.53		
Angrier than willing to admit	.69	.63	−.11	−.12	.59	.52		
Secretly critical of others	.69	.58	−.04	−.02	.59	.47		
Boil inside, don't show it	.68	.66	.09	.17	.56	.51		
Harbor grudges	.67	.71	−.06	−.12	.58	.60		
Keep things in	.61	.61	.11	.08	.49	.50		
Irritated more than others are aware	.60	.60	−.13	−.16	.50	.50		
Slam doors	.04	−.01	.65	.58			.47	.41
Say nasty things	.04	−.11	.64	.67			.49	.53
Make sarcastic remarks	.00	−.12	.63	.55			.46	.41
Argue with others	.06	.06	.61	.59			.46	.45
Lose my temper	−.04	−.01	.59	.72			.42	.57
Strike out at whatever in-furiates me	−.05	−.10	.53	.49			.39	.37
Express my anger	.15	.17	.49	.48			.37	.37
If someone annoys me, I tell them how I feel	−.05	−.11	.44	.68			.32	.48
Control my temper	.52	.44	.43	.50				
Keep my cool	.48	.41	.39	.41				
Calm down faster	.46	.37	.17	.32				
Make threats	−.02	−.15	.44	.46				
Eigenvalues/Alphas	4.53	3.97	3.13	3.55	.84	.81	.73	.75

*Only correlations of .30 or greater are reported.

sons who express anger toward other persons or objects in the environment have somewhat lower BP. However, examination of the scatter plot of the score distributions for the anger and BP measures suggested that the relationships between these measures were curvilinear, that is, moderate levels of anger expression had no more influence on BP than low levels, whereas high levels of anger expression, especially holding anger in, seemed to have a strong impact on BP.

In order to further clarify the nature of the relationship between anger-in and BP, Johnson (1984) divided his subjects into five subgroups on the basis of their AX/In scores. The relationship between SBP and anger-in is shown in Figure 5.1. As may be noted, SBP was substantially higher for students of both sexes who had the highest Anger/In scores, than for students who were low on anger-in, and males were consistently higher than females at every level of the anger-in variable. Moreover, the SBP for the males began to increase at a lower level of anger-in than for the females.

A similar procedure was used to evaluate differences in BP as a function of anger-out (Johnson, 1984; Spielberger et al., 1985). Students with higher AX/Out scores were consistently somewhat lower in SBP, and there was also a trend for lower DBP to be associated with higher AX/Out scores. In contrast to the finding that males were consistently higher than females in SBP, the females were consistently higher than the males in DBP.

Spielberger and co-workers (1985, p. 22) report correlations of the AX Scale with other personality traits that provide evidence of convergent and divergent validity. The correlations of the AX subscales with the STPI trait and state curiosity subscales were essentially zero. Small but significant correlations of the AX subscales with trait anxiety, for both males and females, ranging from .24 to .30, suggested that persons who were high in anger expression and/or suppression were likely to experience anxiety more often than persons with low scores on these measures. The small positive correlations of the AX/In subscale with S-Anxiety suggested that students who tend to suppress their anger were somewhat more anxious in the testing situation.

Pape (1986) used scenes depicting anger-provoking situations to evaluate the emotional reactions and anger coping strategies of university students who differed in anger expression. She administered the AX Scale to 367 undergraduates to identify students who typically either expressed anger in agressive behavior or suppressed their anger. A sample of 28 expressors (high AX/Out, low AX/In scores) and 30 suppressors (low AX/Out, high AX/In scores) were selected to participate in an anger imagery task. Measures of state anger (S-Anger), state anxiety (S-Anxiety), and "predicted anger coping strategy" were completed following each imagery scene. Expressors and suppressors did not differ in S-Anger or S-Anxiety, but expressors were more likely to predict that they would openly express in responding to the imagery scenes, whereas suppressors were more likely to predict that they would suppress their anger. Pape also reported that AX/In and AX/Out

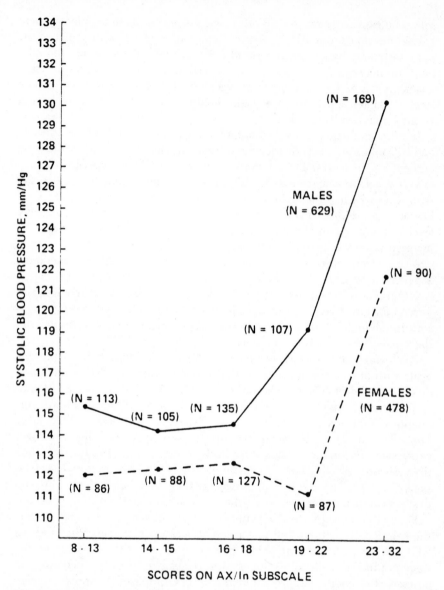

Figure 5.1. Mean systolic blood pressure for five groups of male and female high school students with increasing suppressed anger as measured by scores on the AX/In subscale. This figure is reprinted from "The experience and expression of anger: Construction and validation of an anger expression scale" by C.D. Spielberger and colleagues in *Anger and Hostility in Cardiovascular and Behavioral Disorders*, M.A. Chesney and R.H. Rosenman (Eds.), 1985, New York: Hemisphere Publishing Corporation. Reprinted with permission of the publisher.

scores were not significantly related to social desirability, as measured by the Crowne-Marlowe (1964) scale.

Deffenbacher, Story, Stark, Hogg, and Brandon (1987) used the AX Scale to compare the efficacy of two types of behavioral interventions for anger reduction. Introductory psychology students were selected for this study who: (a) scored in the upper 25% on the STPI T-Anger Scale (scores 22); (b) described themselves as having anger problems; and (c) volunteered to participate in the study when contacted by phone. Approximately equal numbers of men and women were randomly assigned to cognitive-relaxation therapy (CRT), social skills training (SST), and no-treatment control conditions. Both treatment groups showed significant anger reduction, compared with the control condition, and did not differ from one another. At post-treatment and in a 5-week follow-up assessment, both treatment groups were also significantly lower than the no-treatment control group in T-Anger and in the tendency to express and suppress anger as measured by the AX/In and AX/Out Scales.

Williams and Jenkins (1986) used the AX Scale and the STPI S-Anger and T-Anger scales to examine relations of state and trait anger and anger expression with assertiveness and Type-A behavior in 249 undergraduate psychology students. Subjects in the upper and lower extremes of the score distribution (scores < 5, > 12) of the adaption of the Jenkins Activity Survey for college students (Glass, 1977) were classified as Type A and Type B, respectively. Type As scored significantly higher than Type Bs on T-Anger and AX/Out, but did not differ from Type Bs in AX/In. Assertiveness correlated positively and significantly with AX/Out scores ($r = .34, p < .001$), and was negatively correlated with AX/In ($r = -12, p < .01$). Additionally, findings for the Anger EXpression Scale indicated that Type As experience more anger and express anger more often than Type Bs. Type As also rated themselves as more assertive and expressed anger significantly more often than Type Bs, who rated themselves as less assertive and reported that they expressed anger less often.

The Control of Anger

The need to control anger is an important facet of the Type-A behavior pattern. According to Glass (1977), Type-A persons endeavor to gain and maintain control over their environment and continue to try to dominate even after it becomes clear that a situation is unmanageable. While Type As are relatively successful in their efforts to master their environment, if they are frustrated in gaining or maintaining control, they generally experience anger. Whether the anger is expressed in hostile and aggressive behavior or suppressed (Jenkins et al., 1978), the Type A's ability to maintain control is diminished.

The Type A's need to dominate and control and his resistance to being controlled by others have long been recognized. But these needs have been documented in only one study (Burke, 1982), in which the results suggested that Type As endeavor to control their environment and resent others' efforts to dominate them. It should be noted, however, that control was measured in this study by the FIRO-B (Ryan, 1977), which assesses a general desire to control or be controlled. In order to evaluate how Type As manage anger, a valid measure of anger control is needed.

The first step in developing a measure of anger control was to assemble a pool of items with appropriate content. Dictionary definitions of "control" and idioms pertaining specifically to the control of anger were consulted in writing these items. Using the three anger control items from the 20-item AX Scale as a guide, 17 additional items were written. The 17 new anger control items were administered to 409 undergraduates enrolled in introductory psychology classes, along with the 20-item AX Scale, which included the 3 original AX/Con items. Separate principal components factor analyses of the 20 anger control items were carried out for males and females.

The results of these analyses suggested that there was one large anger control (Anger/Con) factor and several very small factors. Items with the strongest loadings on the Anger/Con factor for both males and females were selected for the 8-item AX/Con subscale. Two of the three original AX Scale anger control items were among the items with the highest loadings on the Anger/Con factor. The third item, "I calm down faster than most other people," was also included in the AX/Con subscale to provide continuity with the original AX Scale, even though the loadings of this item on the Anger/Con factor were somewhat lower than those of the other items. In order to confirm the independence of the Anger/Con factor, the final set of 24 items, which included the 8-item AX/Con, AX/Out and AX/In subscales, were factored, separately for males and females. An Anger/Con factor, comprised of all 8 AX/Con items, was the strongest factor to emerge in these analyses. The salient loadings of the 24 AX items on the Anger/Con, Anger/Out, and Anger/In factors are reported in Table 5.2.

Krasner (1986) administered the 24-item AX Scale, the STPI T-Anger Scale and two measures of the TABP—the JAS Form T (Jenkins, Rosenman, & Zyzanski, 1974; Glass, 1977) and the Bortner (1969) Rating Scale—to 409 undergraduate students. Each student was classified as Type A or Type B, depending on whether he/she scored above or below the sample median for each TABP measure. In general, the relationships of the TABP with the STPI measures were similar for the JAS and the Bortner Scale, but were much stronger with the Bortner Scale. Based on the JAS classification, Type-A students scored significantly higher than Type-B students on T-Anger, but no differences were found between these groups on the AX Scales.

When classified on the basis of their scores on the Bortner Scale, the Type-A students scored significantly higher than Type-B students on the T-Anger Scale and the AX/Out subscale, and significantly lower on AX/Con. Significant negative correlations were found between AX/Con and T-Anger for both males ($r = -.64$) and females ($r = -.55$); AX/Con scores also corre-

Table 5.2. Factor Loadings and Alpha Coefficients for the AX Anger/Control, Anger/Out and Anger/In Subscales for College Students

Item Content	Anger/Control M	Anger/Control F	Anger/Out M	Anger/Out F	Anger/In M	Anger/In F
Keep my cool	.76	.73				
Control my behavior	.75	.69				
Control angry feelings	.74	.71	−.33			
Tolerant and under-standing	.68	.69				
Patient with others	.65	.63				
Control my temper	.63	.63	−.41	−.40		
Calm down faster	.57	.52				
Stop myself from losing my temper	.56	.62				
Slam doors	−.35		.32	.49		
Make sarcastic remarks			.67	.52		
Say nasty things	−.32	−.36	.65	.57		
If someone annoys me, I tell them how I feel			.64	.66	−.34	
Express my anger	−.31		.59	.67		
Lose my temper	−.53	−.01	.56	.53		
Strike out at whatever in-furiates me	−.31		.53	.56		
Argue with others			.50	.61		
Irritated more than others are aware					.68	.73
Boil inside, don't show it					.68	.64
Harbor grudges					.68	.62
Angrier than willing to admit					.65	.68
Withdraw from people					.63	.56
Pout or sulk		(−.29)			.53	(.28)
Keep things in			−.33	−.38	.51	.62
Secretly critical of others					.42	.51
Eigenvalues	6.31	6.14	3.20	3.07	1.49	1.52
Alpha coefficients	.85	.84	.75	.77	.73	.74

lated negatively with AX/Out for both sexes ($r = -.59$ for males; $-.58$ for females). Correlations of AX/In scores with AX/Out and AX/Con scores were essentially zero for both sexes. The independence of the AX/In and AX/Out subscales has been consistently demonstrated in previous research (Pollans, 1983; Spielberger et al., 1985).

Solomon (1987) administered the AX Scale and the STPI T-Anger Scale to more than 400 undergraduate students, along with two new experimental scales: The Rationality/Emotional-Defensiveness (R/ED) Scale and the Hopelessness/Depression (H/D) Scale. The R/ED Scale assesses the defensive use of rationality to deny and/or repress feelings; the H/D Scale measures the extent to which specific events or experiences result in chronic feelings of hopelessness and depression. These scales were derived from questionnaires developed by Grossarth-Maticek and his colleagues (e.g., Grossarth-Maticek, Kanazir, Vetter, & Schmidt, 1983) to assess psychosocial risk factors in prospective studies of heart disease and cancer.

Significant positive correlations of the AX/Con subscale with the R/ED Scale ($r = .58$ for males, .57 for females) reported by Solomon suggested that individuals who invested a great deal of energy in controlling the expression of anger were also more likely to use over-rationality, repression, and denial as defenses for controlling their emotions. Significant negative correlations of the R/ED Scale with the T-Anger and AX/Out subscales suggested that students who used over-rationality as a defense in repressing and denying angry feeling experienced and expressed relatively little anger. Significant positive correlations of the T-Anger and AX/In subscales with the H/D Scale suggested that students who experienced more anger, and attempted to cope with anger by suppressing it, felt more hopeless and depressed.

Although the AX Scale was only recently developed, empirical findings linking AX/In and AX/Out to hypertension and the Type-A behavior pattern are encouraging. Johnson (1984) found that high school students with high AX/In scores had higher blood pressure and those with high AX/Out scores had lower BP, than students with low AX/In scores. Type-A college students were found to have higher AX/Out scores than Type Bs (Williams & Jenkins, 1986). Krasner (1986) replicated this finding, and also reported that Type As were higher in T-Anger and had lower AX/Con scores than Type Bs, suggesting that Type As experience more anger and are less effective in controlling it. Solomon (1987) has recently reported that college students who were high on AX/Con and low on AX/Out had higher scores on a measure of emotional defensiveness that had predicted morbidity and mortality for both heart disease and cancer in a prospective study. She also found that students with high AX/In scores were more likely to report prolonged periods of hopelessness and depression.

Summary and Conclusions

There is a great deal of conceptual ambiguity in current theoretical interpretations of anger, hostility, and aggression, and in the methods by which they are measured. On the basis of a review of the research literature, it was concluded that these constructs refer to overlapping phenomena, which we have collectively labeled the AHA! Syndrome. Mounting evidence implicating the AHA! Syndrome in the etiology and pathogenesis of essential hypertension and coronary heart disease calls attention to the critical need to develop objective, reliable, and valid measures of the components of this syndrome.

Because the concept of anger is both more fundamental and simpler than hostility and aggression, anger is at the core of the AHA! Syndrome. Anger has been defined as an emotional state that consists of feelings of irritation, annoyance, fury, and rage, with concommitant activation or arousal of the autonomic nervous system. In the assessment of anger, it is imperative to distinguish, conceptually and empirically, between the intensity of the experience of anger as an emotional state (S-Anger) and individual differences in anger-proneness as a personality trait (T-Anger). It is also essential to differentiate between the experience of angry feelings and how these feelings are expressed.

Three anger scales, reported in the literature in the early 1970s, were briefly reviewed, and a scale recently developed to measure angry feelings, the *State-Trait Anger Scale*, was also described. Research on anger expression was examined and the construction of a self-report, psychometric instrument, the *Anger EXpression* (AX) Scale, was considered in some detail. A major part of the chapter was devoted to examining the psychometric properties of the AX Scale and the validity of its subscales for measuring suppressed anger (anger-in), anger expressed toward other people or objects in the environment (anger-out), and anger control.

The results of several recent studies in which the AX Scale was used to measure anger expression were reported. In these studies, higher scores on the AX/In subscale were related to elevated blood pressure, lack of assertiveness, and reports of prolonged periods of hopelessness and depression. Individuals with high scores on the AX/Out subscale had slightly lower BP, were more assertive, and more likely to be classified as Type A. Preliminary findings with the recently developed AX/Con subscale indicated that college students with high scores were less likely to be classified as Type A, experienced anger less frequently, and were less likely to engage in aggressive behavior. However, they were more likely to use denial and repression as defenses against unacceptable anger impulses. A study in which the AX Scale was used as an outcome measure to evaluate the effectiveness of anger-reduction treatment programs was also reviewed.

References

Alexander, F.G. (1939). Emotional factors in essential hypertension: A tentative hypothesis. *Psychosomatic Medicine, 1,* 175–179.

Alexander, F.G., & French, T.M. (Eds.). (1948). *Studies in psychosomatic medicine: An approach to the cause and treatment of vegetative disturbances.* New York: Ronald.

Averill, J.R. (1982). *Anger and aggression: An essay on emotion.* New York: Springer-Verlag.

Berkowitz, L. (1962). *Aggression: A social psychological analysis.* New York: McGraw-Hill.

Biaggio, M.K., Supplee, K., & Curtis, N. (1981). Reliability and validity of four anger scales. *Journal of Personality Assessment, 45,* 639–648.

Bortner, R.W. (1969). A short rating scale as a potential measure of pattern A behavior. *Journal of Chronic Diseases, 22,* 87–91.

Burke, R.J. (1982). Interpersonal behavior and coping styles of Type A individuals. *Psychological Reports, 51,* 971–977.

Buss, A.H. (1961). *The psychology of aggression.* New York: John Wiley & Sons.

Buss, A.H., & Durkee, A. (1957). An inventory for assessing different kinds of hostility. *Journal of Consulting Psychology, 21,* 343–349.

Caine, T.M., Foulds, G.A., & Hope, K. (1967). *Manual of the hostility and direction of hostility questionnaire (HDHQ).* London: University of London Press.

Cook, W.W., & Medley, D.M. (1954). Proposed hostility and pharisaic-virtue scales for the MMPI. *The Journal of Applied Psychology, 38,* 414–418.

Crowne, D.P., & Marlowe, D. (1964). *The approval motive.* New York: John Wiley & Sons.

Deffenbacher, J.L., Story, D.A., Stark, R.S., Hogg, J.A., & Brandon, A.D. (1987). Cognitive-relaxation and social skills interventions in the treatment of general anger. *Journal of Counseling Psychology, 34,* 171–176.

Dembroski, T.M., MacDougall, J.M., Williams, R.B., & Haney, T.L. (1984). Components of Type A, hostility, and anger-in: Relationship to angiographic findings. *Psychosomatic Medicine, 47,* 219–233.

Diamond, E.L. (1982). The role of anger and hostility in essential hypertension and coronary heart disease. *Psychological Bulletin, 92,* 410–433.

Dunbar, H.F. (1943). *Psychosomatic diagnosis.* New York: Hoeber.

Esler, M., Julius, S., Zweifler, A., Randall, O., Harburg, E., Gardiner, H., & De-Quattro, V. (1977). Mild high-renin essential hypertension. *The New England Journal of Medicine, 296,* 405–411.

Evans, D.R., & Stangeland, M. (1971). Development of the reaction inventory to measure anger. *Psychological Reports, 29,* 412–414.

Feshbach, S. (1964). The function of aggression and regulation of aggressive drive. *Psychological Review,* 257–272.

Friedman, M., & Rosenman, R.H. (1959). Association of specific overt behavior pattern with blood and cardiovascular findings. *Journal of the American Medical Association, 169,* 1286–1296.

Friedman, M., & Rosenman, R.H. (1974). *Type A behavior and your heart.* Greenwich, CT: Fawcett.

Funkenstein, D.H., King, S.H., & Drolette, M.E. (1954). The direction of anger during a laboratory stress-inducing situation. *Psychosomatic Medicine, 16,* 404–413.

Gentry, W.D. (1972). Biracial aggression: I. Effect of verbal attack and sex of victim. *The Journal of Social Psychology, 88,* 75–82.

Gentry, W.D., Chesney, A.P., Gary, H.G., Hall, R.P., & Harburg, E. (1982). Habitual anger-coping styles: I. Effect on mean blood pressure and risk for essential hypertension. *Psychosomatic Medicine, 44,* 195–202.

Gentry, W.D., Chesney, A.P., Hall, R.P., & Harburg, E. (1981). Effect of habitual anger-coping pattern on blood pressure in black/white, high/low stress area respondents. *Psychosomatic Medicine, 43,* 88.

Glass, D.C. (1977). *Behavior patterns, stress and coronary disease.* Hillsdale, NJ: Lawrence Erlbaum Associates.

Grossarth-Maticek, R., Kanazir, D.T., Vetter, H., & Schmidt, P. (1983). Psychosomatic factors involved in the process of carcinogenesis: Preliminary results of the Yugoslav Prospective Study. *Psychotherapy and Psychosomatics, 40*, 191–210.

Harburg, E., Blakelock, E.H., & Roeper, P.J. (1979). Resentful and reflective coping with arbitrary authority and blood pressure: Detroit. *Psychosomatic Medicine, 3*, 189–202.

Harburg, E., Erfurt, J.C., Chape, C., Schull, W., & Schork, M.A. (1973). Socio-ecological stressor areas and black-white blood pressure: Detroit. *Journal of Chronic Diseases, 26*, 596–611.

Harburg, E., & Hauenstein, L. (1980). Parity and blood pressure among four race-stress groups of females in Detroit. *American Journal of Epidemiology, 111*, 356–366.

Harburg, E., Schull, W.J., Erfurt, J.C., & Schork, M.A. (1970). A family set method for estimating heredity and stress-I. *Journal of Chronic Diseases, 23*, 69–81.

Jenkins, C.D., Rosenman, R.H., & Zyzanski, S.J. (1974). Prediction of clinical coronary heart disease by a test for the coronary-prone behavior pattern. *New England Journal of Medicine, 290*, 1271–1275.

Jenkins, C.D., Zyzanski, S.J., & Rosenman, R.H. (1978). Coronary-prone behavior: One pattern or several? *Psychosomatic Medicine, 40*, 25–43.

Johnson, E.H. (1984). *Anger and anxiety as determinants of elevated blood pressure in adolescents.* Unpublished doctoral dissertation, University of South Florida, Tampa.

Krasner, S.S. (1986). *Anger, anger control & the coronary prone behavior pattern.* Unpublished master's thesis, University of South Florida, Tampa.

Matthews, K.A., Glass, D.C., Rosenman, R.H., & Bortner, R.W. (1977). Competitive drive, Pattern A, and coronary heart disease: A further analysis of some data from the Western Collaborative Group Study. *Journal of Chronic Diseases, 30*, 489–498.

Novaco, R.W. (1975). *Anger control: The development and evaluation of an experimental treatment.* Lexington, MA: D.C. Heath.

Pape, N. (1986). *Emotional reactions and anger coping strategies of anger suppressors and expressors.* Unpublished doctoral dissertation, University of South Florida, Tampa.

Pollans, C.H. (1983). *The psychometric properties and factor structure of the Anger EXpression (AX) Scale.* Unpublished master's thesis, University of South Florida, Tampa.

Rosenzweig, S. (1976). Aggressive behavior and the Rosenzweig picture frustration study. *Journal of Clinical Psychology, 32*, 885–891.

Rosenzweig, S. (1978). *The Rosenzweig Picture-Frustration (P-F) Study basic manual and adult form supplement.* St. Louis: Rana.

Ryan, L.R. (1977). *Clinical interpretation of the FIRO-B.* Palo Alto, CA: Consulting Psychologists Press, Inc.

Schachter, S. (1971). *Emotions, obesity and crime.* New York: Academic.

Schultz, S.D. (1954). A differentiation of several forms of hostility by scales empirically constructed from significant items on the MMPI. *Dissertation Abstracts, 17*, 717–720.

Siegel, S. (1956). The relationship of hostility to authoritarianism. *Journal of Abnormal and Social Psychology 52*, 368–373.

Solomon, E.P. (1987). *An examination of personality characteristics and coping mechanisms identified as Putative Risk Factors.* Unpublished master's thesis, University of South Florida, Tampa.

Spielberger, C.D. (1979). *Preliminary manual for the State-Trait Personality Inventory (STPI).* Tampa, FL: University of South Florida, Human Resources Institute.

Spielberger, C.D. (1980). *Preliminary manual for the State-Trait Anger Scale (STAS).*

Tampa, FL: University of South Florida, Human Resources Institute.

Spielberger, C.D. (1983). *Manual for the State-Trait Anxiety Inventory*. Palo Alto, CA: Consulting Psychologists Press.

Spielberger, C.D. (in press). *Manual for the State-Trait Anger Expression Scale (STAXI)*. Odessa, FL: Psychological Assessment Resources, Inc.

Spielberger, C.D., Gorsuch, R.L., & Lushene, R.E. (1970). *Manual for the State-Trait Anxiety Inventory*. Palo Alto, CA: Consulting Psychologists Press.

Spielberger, C.D., Jacobs, G., Russell, S., & Crane, R. (1983). Assessment of anger: The State-Trait Anger Scale. In J.N. Butcher & C.D. Spielberger (Eds.), *Advances in personality assessment*, Vol. 2 (pp. 159–187). Hillsdale, NJ: LEA.

Spielberger, C.D., Johnson, E.H., Russell, S.F., Crane, R.J., Jacobs, G.A., & Worden, T.J. (1985). The experience and expression of anger: Construction and validation of an anger expression scale. In M.A. Chesney & R.H. Rosenman (Eds.), *Anger and hostility in cardiovascular and behavioral disorders* (pp. 5–30). New York: Hemisphere/McGraw-Hill.

Tavris, C. (1982). *Anger, the misunderstood emotion*. New York: Simon & Schuster.

Williams, D.A., & Jenkins, J.D. (1986). Anger, assertiveness and the Type-A Behavior Pattern. Manuscript submitted for publication.

Williams, R.B. Jr., Barefoot, J.C., & Shekelle, R.B. (1985). The health consequences of hostility. In M.A. Chesney & R.H. Rosenman (Eds.), *Anger and hostility in cardiovascular and behavioral disorders* (pp. 173–185). New York: Hemisphere/McGraw-Hill.

Zelin, M.L., Adler, G., & Myerson, P.G. (1972). Anger self-report: An objective questionnaire for the measurement of aggression. *Journal of Consulting and Clinical Psychology, 39*, 340.

6

Social Support, Personality, and Health

Irwin G. Sarason

This review by Sarason vividly describes how certain personal and social factors can influence vulnerability to stress. The focus is upon life events and social support, and how these and other factors may interact to effect health, illness, and happiness. He points out how the original thinking that all life events (positive and negative) contribute to increased vulnerability has been supplanted by recent data indicating serious repercussions for health and adjustment for negative life events, but neutral or positive consequences for positive life events. There follows a review of the issues in the personality and life events-illness relationship that focuses on both individual differences in personality characteristics such as locus of control and sensation seeking, and on the nature of appraisal of life events. Both factors contribute to the determination of the amount of stress that will be experienced by the individual. The majority of the chapter, however, is devoted to the author's research on social support. He sets the background by emphasizing the environmental and individual difference perspectives, both essential to an understanding of the influence of social support upon health. His review of the literature provides both answers and questions, as he probes data related to such diverse things as aging, reproduction and birth complications, immune function, job disruptions, chest pain, and asthma. His own research on the topic is rich and thorough. Through the use of his Social Support Scale, Sarason and his colleagues have provided a clearer picture of the nature of social support and its influence upon the health and illness, not to mention happiness and adjustment, of everyone. As have other authors in this volume, Sarason cautions that we should be cognizant of individual differences—environmental, physiological, and personality— and not be too quick to generalize specific findings to the whole populations. A final emphasis is placed upon the need for research into preventive intervention, as used to enhance social support, and research into the psychophysiology of social support.

—Editor

Most definitions of stress refer to the individual's reactions to situations that pose demands, constraints, or opportunities. Because there are marked differences in how people respond to particular situations, researchers have sought to quantify variables that influence the degree to which they are susceptible to various types of stressors. Whereas some people seem to deteriorate rapidly under severe stress, others show only minimal to moderate deterioration, and still others seem unaffected. There is now considerable evidence that people who in the recent past have had a bunching up of experiences they regard as bad or undesirable are vulnerable to challenges.

Many significant correlations have been reported between assessed life events and illness, although most of them have been small in size. There is growing reason to believe that, in addition to negative life events, a variety of personal and social factors influence vulnerability. One such factor is the person's perception of the availability of social support. This variable may be implicated in reactions to stressors, and may be related to personal adjustment, health, and response to illness. Sizable differences in life events-illness correlations for groups differing in social support have been reported (Sarason, Sarason, Potter, & Antoni, 1985).

This chapter reviews what we know about social support and health, discusses its conceptualization, and suggests some lines of research that might prove productive in future research. To lay the groundwork for these topics, a word should be said about the life stress-illness relationship whose investigation has stimulated much of the interest in social support as a stress moderator.

Stress and Illness

Experience in everyday life suggests that unwanted, undesirable, and threatening events increase personal vulnerability and clinical evidence corroborates this observation (Johnson, 1986). As a consequence, many instruments that assess life events in both adults and children are now available. Early work on these instruments was based on the assumption that negative and positive life events summate to increase vulnerability (Holmes & Rahe, 1967). Recent research has produced instruments that separately assess the occurrence of both negative and positive life events and has shown that, while negative life events have unfortunate consequences for personal adjustment, pleasant events tend, if anything, to have a beneficial effect (Johnson & McCutcheon, 1980; Sarason, Johnson, & Siegel, 1978; Vinokur & Selzer, 1975). Among the conditions to which cumulative negative life changes have been related are cardiac death and myocardial infarction, pregnancy and birth complications, menstrual discomfort, the severity of various types of symptoms, cancer, abdominal pain, and respiratory illness (Johnson, 1986). In addition, there appears to be a relationship between life stress and both athletic injuries and work-related accidents (Bramwell, Wagner, Masuda, &

Holmes, 1975; Levenson, Hirschfeld, Hirschfeld, & Dzubay, 1983). These results are essentially correlational, but they are consistent with the idea that one's experiential history may have a bearing upon vulnerability to illness.

Personality and Life Events-Illness Relationships

That the correlations between life events and health status have not been large is not surprising given that most life events research has neglected personality and social-environmental variables that might influence how the individual responds to demands, constraints, and opportunities. Efforts to clarify the roles of these variables are now visible in the literature and it is widely recognized that the effects of life changes can be moderated by variables outside of and within the individual. Stressors have differential effects on people depending upon (1) their personalities, coping skills, motivations, and past experiences; and (2) their environmental supports, such as, having or not having visits from family members or friends after undergoing surgery. As the moderators of life stress are identified, measured reliably, and included in research designs, increased effectiveness in prediction is likely to result.

Which individuals are most likely to be affected adversely by negative life events? Particular life changes (such as natural disaster) may be imposed on individuals and influence how the changes are dealt with. Identification of those personal attributes that are the most important contributors to how events are processed by people is central in this regard. Locus of control is an illustration of a personality characteristic that differentially influences responses to stress. Johnson and Sarason (1978) found that negative life changes are significantly related to both anxiety and depression, but only for people with an external locus of control. Their results were consistent with the idea that people are more adversely affected by life stress if they perceive themselves as typically having little control over their environment.

Another personality variable, sensation seeking, also seems to serve as a moderator of life stress. Smith, Johnson, and Sarason (1978) examined the relationship between life events as measured by the Life Experiences Survey (LES) (Sarason et al., 1978), sensation seeking, and psychological distress and found that, although subjects who had had many negative life changes and were low in sensation seeking reported relatively high levels of psychological distress, subjects with many negative life changes who were high in sensation seeking did not describe themselves as experiencing distress. These results are consistent with Johnson, Sarason, and Siegel's (1979) finding that individuals low in sensation seeking were more likely to report that they were greatly affected by life changes than were those high in sensation seeking. For low sensation seekers, high negative change scores on the LES were significantly related to measures of anxiety and hostility. The positive change score was unrelated to dependent measures regardless of sensation seeking status.

These findings and others in the literature suggest that it is not life events per se, but how they are appraised, that contributes to stress levels. Illustrative of this point is Pancheri's (1980) study of factors associated with myocardial infarction showing that negative life events and their appraisal as assessed by the LES were associated with the occurrence of infarction. Two factors seemed to be important influences in the appraisal process: the general tendency to react with anxiety to problematic situations and coping styles. There is growing reason to believe that personality characteristics and lifestyles together with social and environmental conditions play roles in health, the sense of well-being, and longevity.

Social Support: Environmental and Individual Differences Perspectives

There are both theoretical and clinical reasons for believing that the support provided by social relationships contributes to positive adjustment and personal development and also provides a buffer against the deleterious effects of stress. Bowlby's (1969, 1980) theory of attachment has greatly stimulated interest in the supportive role of social relationships for both adults and children. The strong, mutually reinforcing ties that soldiers develop with each other contribute to their success and survival. Physicians daily note the salutary effects of their attention and expressed concern on patients' well-being and recovery from illness. Psychotherapists provide their patients with acceptance, in part, because they believe that it has a facilitating effect on the patients' efforts to replace maladaptive with adaptive coping techniques.

Research has revealed sizable differences in life events-illness correlations between groups differing in social support. The differences are particularly large for groups differing in their satisfaction with available support. In one recent comparison, the correlation between negative life events and illness was .21 for subjects high in satisfaction with their social support and .50 for those low in satisfaction (Sarason et al., 1985). This evidence is consistent with the idea that social support plays a health protective role and that how people cognitively appraise the support available to them may have consequences for health.

Social support has been conceptualized both as a characteristic of the environment and an attribute of the person. Because these conceptualizations raise different questions for investigation, I shall review their implications.

Environmental Perspective

The environmental approach to social support focuses attention on the effects of the social milieu on health. Epidemiological and sociological research has reflected the growth of interest in community processes and preventive social actions to ward off psychological disorder and illness (Berkman & Syme,

1979; Caplan, 1974, 1976; Heller, 1979). One of the most influential epi-demiological contributions was that offered by Cassel (1976), who re-viewed evidence from both animal and human research and concluded that a particular aspect of the environment, the presence of other members of the same species, can decrease susceptibility to environmental disease agents. From both a sociological and psychiatric point of view, Caplan (1974, 1976) and his colleagues have focused on the role of support systems in personal adaptation. Caplan is especially interested in support derived from the fami-ly and mutual aid or self-help groups. He has emphasized the roles of reci-procity and mutual feedback in supportive relationships. Weiss (1974) has suggested that there are six major provisions of social relationships: attach-ment, social integration, opportunities for nurturance, reassurance of person-al worth, a sense of reliable alliance, and the availability of guidance.

Individual Differences Perspective

Communities and various types of social organizations can be characterized in terms of their supportiveness, and individuals can also be characterized in terms of the support they receive and how they perceive it. Recognition of social support as an individual difference variable has led to a proliferation of measures intended to assess it. These instruments classify support according to such criteria as the availability and frequency of supportive persons; whether support is provided by family members, friends, or others; whether support is provided within a close or confidant relationship; whether the functions support fulfillment, how the functions are matched with indi-viduals' needs; and the satisfaction with available support. Many researchers consider social support to be a multidimensional concept and include the idea of emotional closeness or intimacy as an important factor.

Social Support and Illness

Although social support has been measured in many different ways, there is a growing body of research evidence suggesting that social ties may have im-portant health implications. Lack of social support, caused either by chronic deficiencies in social skills or sudden losses of loved ones, may significantly influence health status. The moderating effect can be either preventive or rehabilitative. Gore (1978) studied the relationship between social support and workers' health after being laid off and found that a low sense of social support exacerbated illness following the stress of job loss. De Araujo, Van Arsdel, Holmes, and Dudley (1973) reported that asthmatic patients with good social supports required lower levels of medication to produce clinical improvement than did asthmatics with poor social supports. There is much evidence that medical and surgical patients benefit from attention and ex-pressions of friendliness by physicians and nurses (Auerbach & Kilmann,

1977). Sosa, Kennel, and Klaus (1980) found that the presence of a supportive lay person had a favorable effect on length of labor and mother-infant
interaction after delivery. Other researchers have also found links among
social variables, illness, and birth complications (Andrews, Tennant, Hewson, & Schonell, 1978; Cooley & Keesey, 1981).

There is a growing body of evidence suggesting that social resources play
an important role in coronary morbidity and mortality. A 3-year follow-up of
male survivors of initial myocardial infarctions revealed that patients scoring
high on both social isolation and life stress were at elevated risk for sudden
cardiac death as well as for death from all causes (Ruberman, Weinblatt,
Goldberg, & Chaudhary, 1984). In a prospective study of over 7,000 men
evaluating the onset of angina pectoris (chest pain due to insufficient cardiac
blood flow and associated with future myocardial infarction), Medalie and
Goldbourt (1976) found that a wife's love and support was an important
predictor of outcome. Many more patients who had low spouse support experienced more intense angina than did patients with high spouse support.
There is growing evidence suggesting that life stress and low levels of social
support are predictive of all-cause mortality, including coronary heart
disease-related deaths. Interestingly, several animal studies have shown that
disruptions within the social environment and other behavioral manipulations are capable of inducing significant atherosclerotic changes (Manuck,
Kaplan, & Matthews, 1986).

Studies of various bodily systems are being carried out to determine the
role played by social resources in illness. The findings thus far have been
encouraging; for example, several investigations have produced results suggesting that lack of social support may have implications for immune function. Despite many methodological biases and limitations, evidence of an
association between conjugal bereavement and elevated risk of death is growing (Levav, 1982). Bartrop, Luckhurst, Lazarus, Kiloh, and Penny, (1977),
and more recently Schleifer, Keller, Camerino, Thorton, and Stein (1983),
have presented evidence suggesting that loss or anticipated loss of a loved
one may deleteriously affect humoral and cell-mediated immunity. Although
the sample size was small, Monjan's (1983) study suggests that immune
changes under stress do not occur uniformly but, rather, vary with the
personal characteristics of the people who experience stress. Monjan found
that individuals who lacked a confidant and had small social networks
showed depressed responses to mitogens 3 months following the death of a
spouse.

The importance of social networks in relation to immune function is suggested by a series of studies conducted by Kiecolt-Glaser, Garner, and colleagues (1984), and Kiecolt-Glaser, Speicher, and colleagues (1984), which
demonstrated interactions among life stress, self-reported loneliness, symptoms, and immune changes. In their studies of medical students, they found
that two groups are especially susceptible to immune system changes: those
who experience high levels of life stress associated with taking tests and ex-

aminations and those with self-perceived social network deficiencies. Similar results with regard to social networks were obtained with psychiatric in-patients. Research on the complex interactions between psychological and social factors that may enhance or diminish psychobiological adaptation and the physiological mediating mechanisms are clearly fertile and important areas.

Adjustment to Illness

A number of studies have explored the possibility that social support is an asset in recovery from illness. The evidence suggests that people with satisfying social networks are more likely to make better adjustments to illness and disability than people lacking in social support. Support for this conclusion comes from research showing that social support is related to adjustment to spinal cord injury (Warner, Bowers, Rounds, & Kauppl, 1986; Schulz & Decker, 1985), acute coronary disease (Mallick, 1985) and Type II diabetes (Heitzmann & Kaplan, 1984). Illustrative of the role of social support in recovery from illness is research on the psychosocial aspects of recovery from coronary heart disease which has shown that long-lasting emotional distress, family problems, and interpersonal conflict at work have negative effects on recovery (Doehrman, 1977). The study of Type II diabetes by Heitzmann and Kaplan (1984) is of particular interest because these researchers found that social support interacted significantly with gender. For females, satisfaction with supportive relationships was associated with control of the diabetes state. On the other hand, satisfaction with supportive relationships was negatively associated with control for males.

Clinical studies of adjustment to illness fall into two groups, those that relate assessed social support to clinical course, and those in which supportive interventions are employed to influence the course. The studies just cited belong to the first group. Examples of the second group are studies in which mutual aid and support groups are used to facilitate adjustment either for people with disorders or for their family members. These types of interventions seem to have beneficial effects—for example, support groups have proven helpful in lessening the symptoms of genital herpes patients and epilepsy patients (Droge, Arntson, & Norton, 1986; Manne, Sandler, & Zautra, 1986).

Special Populations and Problems

The literature contains a growing number of studies of special populations and clinical problems. For example, there is growing interest in the possibility that psychosocial factors may play important roles in reproductive failure. The presence or absence of social support may be an important factor in reproductive outcomes (Wasser & Isenberg, in press).

Studies of the health status of the elderly illustrate interest in social support as it applies to targeted segments of the population. Although the health of the elderly and how long they live are influenced by a variety of factors, studies are now investigating how social support relates to a person's response to the aging process. Later life is marked by a number of unwanted events and there are important questions about how people adjust to them. For example, how do people incorporate personal losses through death into their lives and move forward? In a study of elderly men and women, Colerick (1985) found that coping histories and current social support levels influence the degree to which older people bounce back from personal losses. Thomas, Garry, Goodwin, and Goodwin (1985) studied independent-living elderly men and women and found that social support played an important role in their levels of health. Research is needed to explicate the nature of the relationships among stress, social support, and health outcomes in people such as the elderly, who are at high risk for morbidity. From a preventive standpoint, there is a need for studies of psychosocial factors that might be protective. For example, McIntosh and Shifflett (1984) showed that older people with satisfying social networks have more healthful diets than comparable people with less satisfying social support. The pathways through which social support exerts this type of influence are unclear and merit exploration.

Methodological and Research Needs

Research on social support and health has turned up some promising leads. However, a number of methodological and theoretical advances are needed for further progress. On the dependent variable side, there has often been a lack of comparability of dependent measures in studies dealing with apparently similar problems. In intervention studies, it is important to know at which physical health outcome stage support is provided, the nature of the support, and the outcome. Most of the social support-health research literature has involved cross-sectional designs. Longitudinal studies that provide information about the course of illness and how people adjust to it are sorely needed.

One research topic that is receiving considerable attention is the assessment of social support. How should it be measured? What are its relevant dimensions? Until these types of questions are answered, we will be confronted with a literature of diverse results that are not based on comparable measures. How social support is assessed grows out of (or should grow out of) how it is conceptualized. Unfortunately, there is little agreement on the conceptualization of social support. Many instruments seem to have been developed largely on the basis of common sense and face validity.

In the next section I shall describe a questionnaire I have developed to assess social support, the research in which it has been used, and the nomological network that is emerging from this work. My reason for doing so is not, I hope, simply egotism. The findings of the assessment and experimental studies with the Social Support Questionnaire that I shall describe suggest some lines of empirical and theoretical development that might prove to be productive.

There is growing evidence that how people appraise the support available to them may be even more important than their actual interpersonal contacts (Heller & Swindle, 1983). In retrospect, this seems understandable given that there are individual differences in the need for social contacts and the personal meanings attached to them. Personal appraisals of social support have several aspects: To whom do people feel they can turn for social contact and help? For which kinds of problems? How satisfied are people with what they derive from their interpersonal relationships?

The Social Support Questionnaire

Objective research on social support requires psychometrically sound, well-validated, and convenient indexes. The Social Support Questionnaire (SSQ) (Sarason, Levine, Basham, & Sarason, 1983) is quite reliable and has considerable construct validity. It consists of 27 items including: "Who accepts you totally, including your worst and your best points?"; "Whom could you count on to help you if you had just been fired from your job or expelled from school?"; "Whom do you feel would help if a family member very close to you died?" Subjects respond to these questions by listing the people who provide pertinent support. The SSQ yields two scores. The first one measures the number of available others individuals feel they can turn to in times of need (Number or Perceived Availability score). The second score measures satisfaction with the support perceived to be available (Satisfaction score). This is indicated on a 6-point Likert scale from "very dissatisfied" to "very satisfied." The SSQ takes 15 to 18 minutes to administer and has good internal consistency and test-retest reliability.

The SSQ was factor analytically derived from a large body of items intended to measure the functions served by social networks. Separate factor analyses of the two SSQ scales showed the Number and Satisfaction to be composed of different, unitary dimensions. A large number of data sets have shown only a moderate correlation between the two components, the correlations typically ranging between .30 and .40. Scores on the Number and Satisfaction scales are negatively related to depression and anxiety, as well as to recollections of anxiety in childhood. The Number score is positively related to extraversion, while the Satisfaction score is inversely related to neuroticism as measured by the Eysenck Personality Inventory (EPI) (Eysenck & Eysenck, 1968). Both scores on the SSQ are negatively correlated with the tendency to experience loneliness and neither score is significantly correlated with a social desirability response set. When the SSQ was compared with an extensive structured interview designed to assess socially supportive relationships, the two approaches yielded comparable results (Sarason, Sarason, Shearin, & Pierce, in press).

The Social Support Questionnaire Short Form

Because of the time constraints in many applied settings, a short form of the SSQ has been developed (Sarason, Shearin, Pierce, & Sarason, 1987). It consists of the 6 items that, over several data sets, produced the highest correlations with both the 27-item SSQ scores and the remaining individual SSQ items. The short form has good internal consistency and test-retest reliability as well as a high degree of correlation with the original instrument. Its correlates with personality measures are also very similar to those of the full-scale SSQ. The short form provides a psychometrically acceptable index that can be obtained in 5 minutes or less. As will be discussed later, the content of the six items identified by factor analyses and item analyses has considerable theoretical interest.

A Person × Situation Approach to Social Support

There has been surprisingly little experimental research on social support and the SSQ has probably been used in most of the controlled laboratory studies that have been carried out. Experimental studies are needed in order to explore how social support as a person variable interacts with controlled, well-defined situations to produce meaningful behavioral patterns. Do groups differing in social support differ in their social behavior? Do they respond differently to stressors? Do they respond differently to environmentally provided support? Answers to these questions can provide clues to the construct validity of social support.

Experimental studies of the SSQ show that subjects high in social support are consistently rated as being more attractive, interesting, and socially skilled than are low scorers (Sarason, Sarason, Hacker, & Basham, 1985). They also have higher morale and seem more optimistic about their lives. Low social support is related to an external locus of control, difficulty in persisting on demanding tasks, increased levels of cognitive interference and stress, and relative dissatisfaction with life (Sarason et al., 1983).

Assessed social support interacts with experimentally manipulated support. Lindner, Sarason, and Sarason (in press) have reported a study in which support was defined in two ways: (1) SSQ Satisfaction (SSQS) scores and (2) experimentally manipulated support. The manipulation was the experimenter's offer of help, if needed, to students who were about to work on a problem-solving test that involved writing stories. The task was similar to the Means-Ends Problem-Solving procedure developed by Platt and Spivack (1975). The experimenter told the subjects that she would be available to them to help them should any problems arise while they wrote their stories. This statement followed her reassurance that many people feel uneasy about writing stories and the subjects should not worry if they feel this way. Although no subject actually requested help, those who had low SSQS scores performed significantly better after receiving the experimental support than a comparable group of low SSQS subjects who did not receive it. The performance of low SSQS subjects who were given this intervention, but not those in the control group, performed as well as the high SSQS subjects. The administered support did not influence the performance of the high SSQS subjects. The interaction of assessed and experimentally provided support was clear: administered support was helpful only to the group whose self-assessed support was low.

This interaction provides impetus for further investigation of experimentally manipulated support, particularly with regard to the definition of specific aspects of situations that might have salutary effects on performance. The interaction may have implications for applied studies of human performance and organizational effectiveness, as well as theories of social support. Probably, the crucial ingredient in the experimental support condition used in this study was communication to the subject of empathy and the availability of help should it be needed. These two ingredients are at least potentially present in most situations in which people perform tasks, for example, interactions among co-acting workers.

This experiment's results related to cognitive processes are also of interest. Low SSQS subjects reported devoting more thought to their problem solutions than did high SSQS subjects. There may be important differences in thinking styles of high and low social support subjects. Low social support subjects spend considerable time thinking about problems on which they are working, perhaps to the detriment of their actual performance. This may have been particularly true for the control condition in the experiment just described. Too much conscious preoccupation with certain problems can have a negative effect. For example, ease in driving a car declines with increases in the driver's preoccupation with the specific steps involved in the task. It may be that low social support individuals perceive social situations as more difficult, feel more on the spot in them, and have more self-preoccupying thoughts than those high in social support. More information is needed about the relationship between social support and task-relevant and task-irrelevant cognitive activity. It would be valuable to compare individuals with different levels of assessed support in terms of their movement from thinking about problems to action concerning them.

Supportive manipulations such as those used in this experiment may exert their influence by reducing feelings of impersonality and concerns about the unavailability of people on whom the individual can rely. People with low levels of social support and/or dissatisfaction with the support available to them may have relatively low levels of belief in the interest other people might have in them. The socially isolated individual is, in a sense, more on the spot than the individual who has ties with others (Jones, 1985). Social support manipulations may reduce perceptions of social isolation.

An important question about social support concerns whether its absence is, in a sense, inflicted upon the individual or is a function of personal attributes or lack of social skills, characteristics that either drive other people away or fail to attract them. If social skills are important factors and if these can be identified, then training strategies to help people alter their social interaction patterns may be a useful way of increasing social support and personal happiness (B.R. Sarason et al., 1985).

The social skills of people differing in social support were recently studied in an experiment in which pairs of subjects differing in assessed social support were videotaped, first while they got acquainted and then while discussing how to solve a hypothetical problem about a troublesome roommate. Each subject's social skills were rated by the experimenter on the basis of his initial contact with the subject after the role plays. Ratings of social behavior were also made by the subject, the subject's partner, and independent raters who viewed the videotape. The physical attractiveness of the subjects based on color snapshots was also rated. Each subject completed a social competence questionnaire and was asked to solve interpersonal problems.

B.R. Sarason and colleagues (1985) found that subjects high in self-described social support scored higher than those low in social support on several measures of social skills. This was true with regard to both perceived availability and satisfaction scores. Those low in social support were described by raters as less likable and less effective than subjects with high social support scores. There were high correlations between the subjects' appraisal of their own social competence and the appraisals made by others. These, in turn, were correlated with the subject's competence as measured by knowledge of appropriate solutions to problem situations. These results clearly indicate that individuals' perceptions of their own social skills are similar to the opinions of others about their skill level. Not only did those high and low in social support elicit different responses from others, and have different opinions about their own skills, but they also seemed to have different cognitions while actually in social situations. Those low in social support described themselves as uncomfortable in looking directly at other people, having problems in getting people to notice them, and lacking confidence in their ability to make friends.

The Lindner and co-workers (in press) findings described earlier suggest the possibility that some social vulnerabilities can be reduced or eliminated by specially planned interventions (Rook, 1984). There would seem to be considerable value in studying the roles of assessed and manipulated social support in situations more complex than those in the studies reported here. For example, for certain kinds of stressful jobs, low social support people might have vulnerabilities that would suggest poor prognosis in carrying out assigned tasks. However, it may be possible to arrange situations so as to reduce these vulnerabilities. If social support is a vulnerability factor it is at least one about which something can be done. Further studies involving social support assessment and experimental manipulations could be important, both theoretically and practically. The practical implications would be enhanced if support could be provided in group settings.

A recent experiment used this approach by administering social support to subjects differing in test anxiety. The subjects before performing in an evaluative situation were exposed to several different experimental conditions, either with or without group interaction (Sarason & Turk, 1983). The conditions represented various combinations of approaches that had been found helpful in previous work in improving the performance of high test-anxious subjects. Some subjects received a written summary of useful coping strategies and were instructed to read them and to write about how to deal with test situations. In a second condition, the subjects were given the same summary and asked to discuss the coping strategies. Subjects in a third condition were asked to write essays about problems related to school but not including tests or test-taking. In a fourth condition, subjects held a general discussion concerning their feelings about such school problems. The fifth group served as a control without any intervention. Subjects in all conditions then worked on moderately difficult anagrams. The subjects who had discussed the specific coping strategies in a group setting showed the most improved performance compared to the controls. Presenting the coping strategies in written form had no effect on performance. The freewheeling group discussion improved performance to a limited degree. For high anxious subjects, writing an essay also improved performance but not as much as the group discussion of coping strategies. In general, the facilitative effects of the experimental intervention were greater for high than low test-anxious subjects.

In a testing situation, highly test-anxious individuals are presumably more stressed than low test-anxious individuals. This study demonstrates, just as the Lindner and co-workers study (in press) did, how the provision of a supportive environment or activity might function to protect individuals, especially those who are particularly vulnerable, from the effects of high stress levels. We found that the combination of support from the group and knowledge of coping techniques produced the best performance especially for highly test-anxious subjects. Presentation of coping techniques in written form was not sufficient to facilitate performance. It is possible that this written presentation might not have been emphatic enough to enable subjects to utilize the skills described. More likely, however, the discussion provided validation of the coping strategies and combined emphasis on the particular points with a supportive interaction that also provided suggestions for effective behaviors. The results concerning this discussion stood in contrast to the freewheeling group discussions that frequently brought out gripes, fears, and other negative thoughts and feelings without giving impetus to behavior change. The results confirm the frequent observation of therapists, as well as parents, that a combination of support and coping strategies is much more effective than empathy alone in producing a change in behavior. One of the benefits of studying supportive behaviors in a laboratory setting is the role

experimental manipulations can play in understanding how and why interventions intended to be supportive produce their effects.

What Is Social Support?

Although a considerable amount of evidence relating some aspects of social
support to a variety of outcome variables has been obtained, the theoretical
implications of these findings is obscured by a lack of information on the
comparability of available support measures. We have recently compared
the SSQs of college students with other widely used social support indices to
identify possible commonalities. Our data suggest that in varying degrees,
each of the instruments assesses the extent to which an individual is
accepted, loved, and involved in relationships in which communication is
open (Sarason et al., 1987). Those individuals who currently had relationships involving these qualities were less depressed and lonely and were
more satisfied with current relationships than were those who did not.

There is currently much interest in delineating the functions of social support, and although supportive others certainly provide useful functions, conceptualizing important relationships in functional terms as providing "services" may produce too narrow a focus for investigative efforts in the field of
social support. Problems with the functional approach may arise for several
reasons. Sometimes what is provided, although intended to be helpful, may
not be experienced as appropriate for the person's situation. For instance,
provision of information and instruction for dealing with a problem situation
may result in communicating to the recipient that he or she is inept and
incapable. Provision of a monetary loan, although appropriate to solve an
immediate problem, may result in feelings of dependence or obligation. Even
emotional support intended to be sympathetic or to help the person return to
normal functioning may be experienced as critical or lacking in understanding (Wortman & Lehman, 1985). Perhaps the greatest difficulty with the
functional approach is that the usefulness of support, when only its functional aspect is considered, cannot be effectively evaluated. The support, even if
useful in the immediate situation, may also convey negative messages to the
recipient that relate to personal effectiveness or independence. The receipt of
such support may also engender guilt or unwelcome feelings of indebtedness.

Perhaps a more useful conceptualization of social support involves viewing
an individual as engaging in a number of relationships, each differing in
quality and depth of caring. A supportive relationship involves the communication of acceptance and love. It is this feeling—that we are loved and
valued, that our well-being is the concern of significant others—that is protective. Yet the main effect of these communicated feelings is not to protect
the individuals from possible harm per se, but to foster in supported individuals the feeling that they are worthwhile, capable, and valued members of
a group of individuals and that the resources necessary for the pursuit and

achievement of their goals are available to them, either within themselves or through a combination of their own efforts and those of their significant others.

The function that social support plays in a person's life is quite likely an extension of that played by attachment experiences in childhood. Whereas supportive attachment experiences in childhood foster a sense of personal worth and provide children with a secure base from which to explore their surroundings, supportive relationships in later life maintain and improve the sense that one is valued and loved. This support continues to promote "exploratory behavior" in which, throughout the life span, tasks are undertaken that are meaningful to the individual and are in the pursuit of meaningful goals.

Social support is often communicated through such supportive behaviors as loans of money, advice, and shoulders to cry on. Yet, the offer and receipt of these provisions does not constitute social support. Nor should each of these supportive behaviors be viewed as conceptually distinct categories of support. Individuals who value and care about us are willing to do for us what they can. Although supportive others differ in their ability to provide money or communicate love, knowing that others love us and would willingly do for us what they can is the essence of social support.

This does not mean that sampling the availability of specific supportive acts does not provide us with useful information about social support. It is probably true that certain behaviors are more likely to convey support than are others. To the extent that these behaviors typically reflect the degree to which the individual is cared for, measures of supportive behaviors—either perceived or received—will be measuring social support. Both types of support measures, those that deal with the support perceived to be available and those that deal with support that has been received, have limitations.

In the course of our comparison of social support measures, we have found an interesting sex difference. Scores on measures of received support are probably influenced by the experience of life events; individuals who are currently dealing with stressful life events may be receiving more acts of support than are others. In addition, people who are better able to cope successfully with life events on their own will probably be the recipients of fewer supportive acts than less competent people. On the other hand, perceived support measures assume that the perceived support experienced by individuals is actually available to them. However, available evidence suggests that it is the perception of support, rather than its actual receipt, that is most related to good adjustment. In general, the correlations between measures of social support are stronger for women than men. This may to some extent be an artifact of the item content of the social support indices that have been used. Additionally, it may result from a hesitancy on the part of male subjects to think about or describe themselves in terms of the particular supportive experiences and outcome variables assessed. Sarason and colleagues (1987), examined the items of several support measures and noted a possible bias toward the types of relationships that women are most likely to find support-ive. Although men certainly have a need to be intimate and to confide in someone whom they are assured cares for them, this type of relationship is more characteristic for women. Supportive relationships for men are perhaps more "comradely" relationships that provide them with opportunities to get their minds off their troubles, rather than opportunities for confiding. The open expression of esteem and affection is probably more prevalent in the relationships of women than of men. Men of college age generally appear less likely than women to receive social support from their family members. They are also less likely to endorse items on symptomatology indices because these instruments deal with problems that carry more negative overtones for men than for women.

It must be cautioned that the generalization based on our social support findings across age groups and, perhaps, socioeconomic groups should, at best, be taken as tentative. As Procidano and Heller (1983) and Cutrona (1986) have pointed out, the composition of a person's support network is likely to change over time. Eckenrode (1983) found that women of low socioeconomic status are less able to make use of social support than others. Bearing this caution in mind, our evidence suggests several important im-plications for future research. First, research on social support might profit from investigations that examine the antecedents of adult support networks. Conceptualizing social support as a developmental personality character-istic, rather than as simply an environmental provision, would contribute greatly to current theories of social support. Second, studies investigating social support need to take into account sex differences, response biases, and differences in the behaviors sought in supportive relationships. Third, re-searchers need to recognize that current support indices measure a variety of behaviors that, although often received in the context of supportive relation-ships, are to some extent also received from nonsupportive others. Thus, a person's experience of being loved and accepted may provide the most accurate assessment of the construct.

What is the relationship between feeling loved and accepted and health and what are the mediating processes? Although we cannot yet answer this question, we can point to research approaches that might help us answer it in the forseeable future. I have already mentioned that, in addition to assess-ment and clinical studies, there is a need for controlled experimental in-tervention dealing with the effects of social support. One type of experimental investigation is illustrated by the study of Whitcher and Fisher (1979), in which the subjects were hospitalized surgical patients and the treatment was social support. Social support was defined simply as nurses touching patients according to a prescribed schedule. The manipulation added significantly to both the medical and psychological progress of the patients.

Two types of research would make valuable contributions to our under-standing of the social support-health relationships. One is preventive in-terventions in which health status and psychological adjustment are examined as a function of opportunities for enhanced social support. The other is controlled studies of differences in bodily processes—such as heart rate, blood pressure, and immunocompetence—as a function of assessed and manipulated social support.

References

Andrews, G., Tennant, C., Hewson, D., & Schonell, M. (1978). The relation of social factors to physical and psychiatric illness. *American Journal of Epidemiology, 108*, 27–35.

Auerbach, S.M., & Kilmann, P.R. (1977). Crisis intervention: A review of outcome research. *Psychological Bulletin, 84*, 1189–1217.

Bartrop, R.W., Luckhurst, E., Lazarus, L., Kiloh, L.G., & Penny, R. (1977). Depressed lymphocyte function after bereavement. *Lancet*, 834–836.

Berkman, L.F., & Syme, S.L. (1979). Social networks, host resistance, and mortality: A nine-year follow-up study of Alameda County residents. *American Journal of Epidemiology, 109*, 186–204.

Bowlby, J. (1969). *Attachment*. New York: Basic Books.

Bowlby, J. (1980). *Loss: Sadness and depression*. New York: Basic Books.

Bramwell, S.T., Wagner, N.N., Masuda, N.M., & Holmes, T.H. (1975). Psychosocial factors in athletic injuries. *Journal of Human Stress, 1*, 6–20.

Caplan, G. (1974). *Support, systems and community mental health: Lectures on concept development*. New York: Behavioral Publications.

Caplan, G. (1976). The family as support system. In G. Caplan & M. Killilea (Eds.), *Support systems and mutual help: Multidisciplinary explorations* (pp. 19–36). New York: Grune & Stratton.

Cassel, J. (1976). The contribution of the social environment to host resistance. *American Journal of Epidemiology, 104*, 107–123.

Colerick, E.J. (1985). Stamina in later life. *Social Science Medicine, 21*, 997–1006.

Cooley, E.J., & Keesey, J.C. (1981). Moderator variables in life stress and illness relationship. *Journal of Human Stress, 8*, 35–40.

Cutrona, C.E. (1986). Objective determinants of perceived social support. *Journal of Personality and Social Psychology, 50*, 349–355.

De Araujo, G., Van Arsdel, P.O., Holmes, T.H., & Dudley, D.L. (1973). Life change, coping ability and chronic intrinsic asthma. *Journal of Psychosomatic Research, 17*, 359–363.

Doehrman, S.R. (1977). Psycho-social aspects of recovery from coronary heart disease: A review. *Social Science & Medicine, 11*, 199–218.

Droge, D., Arntson, P., & Norton, R. (1986). The social support function in epilepsy self-help groups. *Small Group Behavior, 17*, 139–163.

Eckenrode, J. (1983). The mobilization of social support: Some individual constraints. *American Journal of Community Psychology, 11*, 509–528.

Eysenck, H.J., & Eysenck, S.B. (1968). *Manual: Eysenck Personality Inventory*. San Diego, CA: Educational and Industrial Testing Service.

Gore, S. (1978). The effects of social support in moderating the health consequences of unemployment. *Journal of Health and Social Behavior, 19*, 157–165.

Heitzmann, C.A., & Kaplan, R.M. (1984). Interaction between sex and social support in the control of Type II diabetes mellitus. *Journal of Consulting and Clinical Psychology, 52*, 1087–1089.

Heller, K. (1979). The effects of social support: Prevention and treatment implications. In A.P. Goldstein & F.H. Kanfer (Eds.), *Maximizing treatment gains* (pp. 353–382). New York: Academic Press.

Heller, K., & Swindle, R.W. (1983). Social networks, perceived social support and coping with stress. In R.D. Felner, L.A. Jason, J. Moritsugu, & S.S. Farber (Eds.), *Preventive psychology: Theory, research and practice in community intervention* (pp. 87–103). New York: Pergamon Press.

Holmes, T.H., & Rahe, R.H. (1967). The social readjustment rating scale. *Journal of Psychosomatic Research, 11*, 213–218.

Johnson, J.H. (1986). *Life events as stressors in childhood and adolescence.* Newbury Park, CA: Sage Publications.

Johnson, J.H., & McCutcheon, S.M. (1980). Assessing life stress in older children and adolescents: Preliminary findings with the Life Events Checklist. In I.G. Sarason & C.D. Spielberger (Eds.), *Stress and Anxiety*, Vol. 7 (pp. 111–125). Washington, DC: Hemisphere Publishing Corporation.

Johnson, J.H., & Sarason, I.G. (1978). Life stress, depression and anxiety: Internal-external control as a moderator variable. *Journal of Psychosomatic Research, 22*, 205–208.

Johnson, J.H., Sarason, I.G., & Siegel, J.M. (1979). Arousal seeking as a moderator of life stress. *Perceptual and Motor Skills, 49*, 665–666.

Jones, W.H. (1985). The psychology of loneliness: Some personality issues in the study of social support. In I.G. Sarason & B.R. Sarason (Eds.), *Social support: Theory, research and applications* (pp. 225–241). Dordrecht, The Netherlands: Martinus Nijhoff Publishers.

Kiecolt-Glaser, J.K., Garner, W., Speicher, C., Penn, G., Holliday, J., & Glaser, R. (1984). Psychosocial modifiers of immunocompetence in medical students. *Psychosomatic Medicine, 46*, 7–14.

Kiecolt-Glaser, J.K., Speicher, C.E., Holiday, J.E., & Glaser, R. (1984). Stress and the transformation of lymphocytes by Epstein-Barr virus. *Journal of Behavioral Medicine, 7*, 1–12.

Levav, I. (1982). Mortality and psychopathology following the death of an adult child: An epidemiological review. *Israel Journal of Psychiatry and Related Science, 19*, 23–38.

Levenson, H., Hirschfeld, M.L., Hirschfeld, A., & Dzubay, B. (1983). Recent life events and accidents: The role of sex differences. *Journal of Human Stress, 9*, 4–8.

Lindner, K.C., Sarason, I.G., & Sarason, B.R. (in press). Assessed life stress and social support and experimentally provided social support. In C.D. Spielberger & I.G. Sarason (Eds.), *Stress and anxiety*, Vol. 11. Washington, DC: Hemisphere Publishing Corporation.

Mallick, M.J. (1985). A community-based support group for families and patients after acute coronary disease. *Public Health Nursing, 2*, 43–50.

Manne, S., Sandler, I., & Zautra, A. (1986). Coping and adjustment to genital herpes: The effects of time and social support. *Journal of Behavioral Medicine, 9*, 163–177.

Manuck, S.B., Kaplan, J.R., & Matthews, K.A. (1986). Behavioral antecedents of coronary heart disease and arteriosclerosis. *Arteriosclerosis, 6*, 2–14.

McIntosh, W.A., & Shifflett, P.A. (1984). Influence of social support systems on dietary intake of the elderly. *Journal of Nutrition for the Elderly, 4*, 5–18.

Medalie, J.H., & Goldbourt, U. (1976). Angina pectoris among 10,000 men: II. Psychosocial and other risk factors as evidenced by a multivariate analysis of a five-year incidence study. *American Journal of Medicine, 60*, 910–921.

Monjan, A.A. (1983). Effects of acute and chronic stress upon lymphocyte blasto-genesis in mice and humans: "Of mice and men." In E.L. Cooper (Ed.), *Stress, immunity, and cancer* (pp. 81–108). New York: Marcel Dekker.

Pancheri, P. (1980). Psycho-neural-endocrinological correlates of myocardial in-farction. Paper presented at NIAS International Conference on Stress and Anxiety, Wassenaar, The Netherlands.

Platt, J.J., & Spivack, G. (1975). *Manual for the Means-Ends Problem-Solving Procedure.* Philadelphia: Hahnemann Community Mental Health Center.

Procidano, M.E., & Heller, K. (1983). Measures of perceived social support from friends and from family: Three validation studies. *American Journal of Community Psychology, 11(1)*, 1–24.

Rook, K.S. (1984). Promoting social bonding: Strategies for helping the lonely and socially isolated. *American Psychologist, 39*, 1389–1407.

Ruberman, W., Weinblatt, E., Goldberg, J.D., & Chaudhary, B.S. (1984). Psycho-social influences on mortality after myocardial infarction. *The New England Journal of Medicine, 311*, 552–559.

Sarason, B.R., Sarason, I.G., Hacker, T.A., & Basham, R.B. (1985). Concomitants of social support: Social skills, physical attractiveness and gender. *Journal of Personality and Social Psychology, 49*, 469–480.

Sarason, B.R., Shearin, E.N., Pierce, G.R., & Sarason, I.G. (1987). Interrelation-ships of social support measures: Theoretical and practical implications. *Journal of Personality and Social Psychology, 52*, 813–832.

Sarason, I.G., Johnson, J.H., & Siegel, J.M. (1978). Assessing the impact of life changes: Development of the Life Experiences Survey. *Journal of Consulting & Clinical Psychology, 46*, 932–946.

Sarason, I.G., Levine, H.M., Basham, R.B., & Sarason, B.R. (1983). Assessing social support: The Social Support Questionnaire. *Journal of Personality and Social Psychology, 44*, 127–139.

Sarason, I.G., Sarason, B.R., Potter, E.H., & Antoni, M.H. (1985). Life events, social support and illness. *Psychosomatic Medicine, 47*, 156–163.

Sarason, I.G., Sarason, B.R., Shearin, E.N., & Pierce, G.R. (1987). A brief measure of social support: Practical and theoretical implications. *Journal of Personal and Social Relationships, 4*, 497–510.

Sarason, I.G., & Turk, S. (1983). *Coping strategies and group interaction: Their function in improving performance of anxious individuals.* Unpublished manuscript, University of Washington, Seattle.

Schleifer, S.J., Keller, S.E., Camerino, M., Thornton, J.C., & Stein, M. (1983). Sup-pression of lymphocyte stimulation following bereavement. *Journal of the American Medical Association, 250*, 374–377.

Schulz, R., & Decker, S. (1985). Long-term adjustment to physical disability: The role of social support, perceived control, and self-blame. *Journal of Personality and Social Psychology, 48*, 1162–1172.

Smith, R.E., Johnson, J.H., & Sarason, I.G. (1978). Life change, the sensation seek-ing motive, and psychological distress. *Journal of Consulting and Clinical Psychology, 46*, 348–349.

Sosa, R., Kennel, J., & Klaus, M. (1980). The effect of a supportive companion on perinatal problems, length of labor and mother-infant interactions. *New England Journal of Medicine, 305*, 597–600.

Thomas, P.D., Garry, P.J., Goodwin, J.M., & Goodwin, J.S. (1985). Social bonds in a healthy elderly sample: Characteristics and associated variables. *Social Science Medicine, 20*, 365–369.

Thomas, P.D., Goodwin, J.M., & Goodwin, J.S. (1985). Effect of social support on stress-related changes in cholesterol level, uric acid level, and immune function in an elderly sample. *American Journal of Psychiatry, 142*, 735–737.

Vinokur, A., & Selzer, M.L. (1975). Desirable versus undesirable life events: Their relationship to stress and mental distress. *Journal of Personality and Social Psychology, 32*, 329–337.

Warner, G.C., Bowers, P.M., Rounds, J.B., & Kauppl, R. (1986). *Social support, stress, and adjustment to spinal cord injury.* Paper presented at the 94th Annual meeting of the American Psychological Association, Washington, DC.

Wasser, S.K., & Isenberg, D.Y. (in press). Reproductive failure among women: Pathology or adaptation? *Journal of Psychomatic Obstetrics and Gynecology.*

Weiss, R.S. (1974). The provisions of social relationships. In Z. Rubin (Ed.), *Doing unto others* (pp. 17–26). Englewood Cliffs, NJ: Prentice-Hall.

Whitcher, S.J., & Fisher, J.D. (1979). Multidimensional reaction to therapeutic touch in a hospital setting. *Journal of Personality and Social Psychology, 37*, 87–96.

Wortman, C.B., & Lehman, D.R. (1985). Reactions to victims of life crisis: Support attempts that fail. In I.G. Sarason & B.R. Sarason (Eds.), *Social support: Theory, research and application* (pp. 463–490). Dordrecht, The Netherlands: Martinus Nijhoff Publishers.

7
Personality and Stress as Causal Factors in Cancer and Coronary Heart Disease

Hans J. Eysenck

In this chapter, Eysenck relates that since the times of Hippocrates and Galen there has been the tradition in medicine that certain personality characteristics are related to specific diseases. For example, the lack of emotional expression and feelings of impotence in the presence of unavoidable stress are characteristics attributed to victims of cancer. Cancer and heart disease are the focus here, as the evidence of consistent but contrasting personality characteristics being related to each is described. Past attempts at research in this area are criticized for their lack of theory, as Eysenck emphasizes the importance of putting forward hypotheses that can be tested, rather than pointing to correlations that cannot be interpreted causally. The bulk of the paper is given over to a description of two large-scale prospective studies, in two different parts of Europe: Crevenka, Yugoslavia and Heidelberg, West Germany. The striking thing about the two studies is the remarkable similarity of the data with relating personality characteristics and cancer/cardiovascular disease. Subjects were divided into four broad categories, the principal ones being Type I (cancer-prone—hopelessness, helplessness, depressive feelings, and repression in the face of stress) and Type II (coronary-prone—responding to stress with emotional expression, anger, irritation, and having unstable emotional relations). The hypothesized relationship was demonstrated. In both samples, Type I subjects were more likely than others to die of cancer, while Type II subjects were more like to suffer mortality due to infarct or stroke. Many other fascinating parallels in these data are described and related to the current known literature on both cancer and cardiovascular disease. In supporting so well some of the traditional beliefs about cancer and coronary disease, these data are both startling and provocative. They provide much needed fuel for future work and an empirical background for future hypothesis testing.

—EDITOR

There is a long tradition in medicine, dating back to Hippocrates and Galen, to the effect that certain diseases are more likely to occur in certain personality types. Cancer, in particular, has been linked over the years with two major personality traits. One of these is *lack of emotional* expression, or actual *emotional repression*. The other is a tendency to develop *feelings of hopelessness and helplessness* in the face of unavoidable stress. In recent years, beginning with the work of Kissen and Eysenck (1962), there has been an increasing tendency to submit these hypotheses, which were developed on a purely observational basis, to a more objective and empirical scrutiny. A detailed survey of the evidence by Eysenck (1985a) has shown that many studies support the proposition that personality is closely linked with cancer, and there is now much evidence to show that similarly, coronary heart disease is linked with personality. The evidence suggests that the personality types prone to cancer and coronary heart disease are quite different, and indeed in many ways the opposite one of the other. Thus aggressiveness is part of the coronary heart disease-prone personality, but if anything, is negatively correlated with cancer proneness. The same seems to be true of anxiety or neuroticism.

Although there is considerable agreement among different studies, most of them suffer from certain weaknesses that make it difficult to accept the conclusions as definitive. Particularly doubtful are studies comparing cancer or cardiovascular diseased patients with patients suffering from other disorders, or with normals; the knowledge of suffering from these diseases may lead to changes in personality that are not causally related to the illness in a prospective sense. Many of the studies, following the Kissen and Eysenck (1962) patern, have looked at patients presenting at the clinic and administering questionnaries *prior* to diagnosis. In this way, all the patients fear that the diagnosis may be of cancer or cardiovascular disease, but none of them know what the diagnosis will be. Comparisions can then be made between those who are found to suffer from cancer or cardiovascular disease, and those who do not. Although this is a superior design, nevertheless prospective studies are of course essential if we are to come to any definitive conclusions.

Another weakness of previous research is the lack of any causal theory. An attempt has been made to supply such a theory (Eysenck, 1983, 1984, 1985b), and will be discussed later on in this chapter. Correlation, however impressive, cannot directly be interpreted in a causal manner, and that makes it all the more important to put forward causal hypotheses which can be experimentally tested.

Details of the several prospective studies, results of which will be reviewed in this chapter, are contained in a series of papers by Grossarth-Maticek (1980) and Grossarth-Maticek and colleagues (1983, 1986). To be discussed are two longitudinal studies, each carried out over a period of 10 years. The first was conducted in Crevenka, a village in Northeastern Yugoslavia, with about 14,000 inhabitants, between 1965 and 1976. The other was conducted in Heidelberg in West Germany, which has about 140,000 inhabitants, between 1972 and 1982. In the Yugoslavian study, which included 1,353 subjects, a random sample of houses was determined, and in each case the oldest inhabitant was studied, provided that he or she was not suffering from cancer, coronary heart disease, or any other serious disorder. In the Heidelberg study a truly random sample of 872 subjects was established—this will be called the "normal" sample. Subjects also nominated people they knew who were stressed, those who by personality, smoking and drinking habits, personal loss, etc. were considered under stress; these form a part of the sample that contained 1,273 subjects. This will be called the "stressed" Heidelberg sample.

At the beginning of the respective time intervals, psychosocial data were collected by means of interviews with standardized questions, and of interviewer ratings. Medical data were also established, including cigarette smoking, drinking, etc. At the end of the 10- or 11-year period, mortality and cause of death were recorded; in the case of the Heidelberg study by a university department completely independent of the investigators.

Two types of analysis were carried out. In the first, derived from the Yugoslav study, a questionnaire containing 109 questions concerning personality was filled in by the subjects at the begining of the study. Scales were derived dealing with questions related to adverse life events or situations leading to lasting hopelessness/helplessness; adverse life events or situations leading to anger and/or hostility and aggression; rationality and anti-emotionality (i.e., the obverse of neuroticism); anxiety; harmonious interpersonal relationships; ignoring signs of illness (lack of hypochondriasis); lack of potential emotional relations; absence of self-reported psychopathological symptoms, especially anxiety; and acquiescence. Quite high correlations were reported with later development of cancer—.59 with hopelessness/helplessness, .51 with rationality/anti-emotionality, .49 with drive for harmony, −.39 with hypochondriasis, etc. (Schmidt, 1984). These correlations are well in line with the theories and observations mentioned above (Eysenck, 1988).

Obviously the various scales are not independent, and it is of some interest to discover to what extent they can be used jointly to arrive at a multiple correlation. Grossarth-Maticek, Kanazir, Schmidt, and Vetter (1982, p. 297) have constructed a path model with cancer as the dependent variable and seven psychosocial scales as the independent variables. The results, in the form of standardized partial regression coefficients are given in Figure 7.1. It will be seem that X_1 (hopelessness) and X_3 (rationality/anti-emotionality) retain their strong positive relationship with cancer incidence, and that X_2 (excitement) retains a marked negative correlation. The other variables have quite low regression coefficients. The explained variance (R^2) for these seven variables is .55, with an error term denoting the unexplained variance of .45;

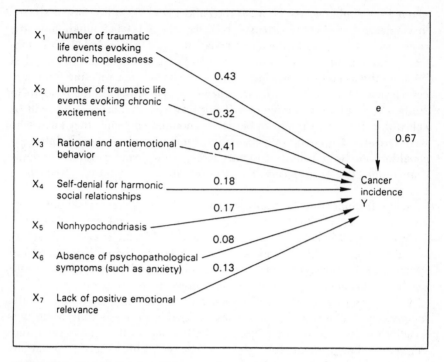

Figure 7.1. Standardized partial regression coefficients in the prediction of cancer.

this is indicated in Figure 7.1 as e (e = R). Actually the R^2 for the first three predictors is equal to .49, so that there is little gained by including X_4, X_5, X_6, and X_7.

An alternative method of looking at personality, integrating the traits studied into a composite personality type has proved even more productive (Grossarth-Maticek, Eysenck, & Vetter, 1987). In order to study the relationship between personality, as established at the beginning of the study, and later mortality, probands were divided into four personality types, type I being (according to theory) cancer-prone, type II coronary heart disease-prone, and types III and IV not prone to either of these two disorders (Eysenck, 1987a). A detailed description of the personality types can be found elsewhere (Grossarth-Maticek et al., 1986). Briefly, the cancer-prone personality type deals with stress through loss of the loved object, or frustrative non-reward by the loved object, with feelings of hopelessness, helplessness, and depression, retains emotional closeness with withdrawing objects, shows a tendency to idealize the withdrawing objects, and represses overt emotional reactions. Type II reacts to stress and frustrative non-reward by chronic irritation and anger, tends to give an extreme evaluation of the disturbing objects, and fails to establish stable emotional relations. Types III and IV, although different, avoid these extreme reactions.

Table 7.1. Mortality and Causes of Deaths in the Sample

	Yugoslavia	Heidelberg	
		Normal	Stressed
Alive	750 = 55.4%	773 = 88.6%	566 = 54.3%
Died from			
cancer	166 = 12.3%	29 = 3.3%	199 = 19.1%
infarct or stroke	156 = 11.5%	27 = 3.1%	120 = 11.5%
other causes	281 = 20.8%	43 = 4.9%	157 = 15.1%
Total: successfully followed-up	1,353	872	1,042 (without therapy and control groups)

Table 7.2. Mortality and Causes of Death by Psychosocial Type: Yugoslavia

Type	Alive	Cancer	Infarct or Stroke	Other	Total
I	76 = 25.1%	140 = 46.2%	25 = 8.3%	62 = 20.5%	303
II	101 = 29.8%	19 = 5.6%	99 = 29.2%	120 = 35.4%	339
III	129 = 59.4%	4 = 1.8%	20 = 9.2%	64 = 29.5%	217
IV	438 = 90.9%	3 = 0.6%	8 = 1.7%	33 = 6.8%	482
Unclassified	6	0	4	2	12
Total	750 = 55.4%	166 = 12.3%	156 = 11.5%	281 = 20.8%	1353

χ^2 (Mantel-Haenszel, controlling for sex and age) = 661, df = 9

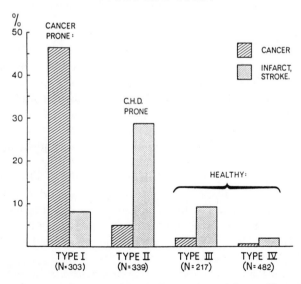

Figure 7.2. Mortality and causes of deaths by psychosocial type: Yugoslavian study.

Table 7.3. Mortality and Causes of Deaths by Psychosocial Type: Heidelberg Normal Sample

Type	Alive	Cancer	Infarct or stroke	Other	Total
I	78 = 71.6%	19 = 17.4%	2 = 1.8%	10 = 9.2%	109
II	109 = 64.1%	10 = 5.9%	23 = 13.5%	28 = 16.5%	170
III	185 = 98.4%	0	1 = 0.5%	2 = 1.1%	188
IV	387 = 99.0%	0	1 = 0.3%	3 = 0.8%	391
Unclassified	14	0	0	0	14
Total	773 = 88.6%	29 = 3.3%	27 = 3.1%	43 = 4.9%	872

HEIDELBERG STUDY
(normal group)

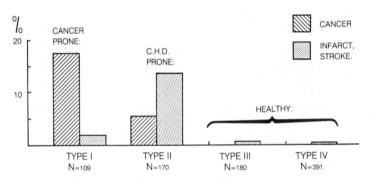

Figure 7.3. Mortality and causes of deaths by psychosocial type: Heidelberg normal sample.

Table 7.1 shows the mortality and causes of death in the various samples. As will be seen, the proportion still alive is of course much larger in the Heidelberg "normal" study, because in the Yugoslavian study the sample was much older, and in the Heidelberg "stressed" sample the stress would theoretically have led to a greater number of deaths. As will be seen, the death rate is almost equal for the Yugoslavian and the Heidelberg "stressed" sample.

Table 7.2 shows the mortality and causes of death by personality type in the Yugoslavian study. The most important part of the table is that relating to the large number of deaths from cancer in type I, and the large number of deaths from infarct or stroke in type II, as compared with each other and with types III and IV. Figure 7.2 shows in diagrammatic form the striking differences between the types.

Table 7.3 and Figure 7.3 perform the same service for the normal Heidel-

Table 7.4. Mortality and Causes of Deaths by Psychosocial Type: Heidelberg Stress Sample

Type	Alive	Cancer	Infarct or stroke	Other	Total
I	188 = 38.1%	188 = 38.4%	34 = 7.0%	79 = 16.2%	489
II	148 = 47.9%	7 = 2.3%	86 = 27.8%	69 = 22.0%	309
III	153 = 92.7%	4 = 2.4%	0	8 = 4.8%	165
IV	71 = 97.3%	0	0	2 = 2.7%	73
Unclassified	6	0	0	0	6
Total	566 = 54.3%	199 = 19.1%	120 = 11.5%	157 = 15.1%	1,042

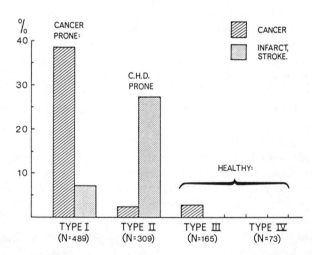

Figure 7.4. Mortality and causes of deaths by psychosocial type: Heidelberg stress sample.

berg sample. There are of course many fewer deaths in this sample, but the difference between the types is very much in line with the results of the Yugoslavian study.

Finally, Table 7.4 and Figure 7.4 show the results from the Heidelberg stressed group. The data are very similar to those from the Yugoslav study, and it may be said that there are now three studies, constituting an original study and two replications, which indicate a close relationship between personality type, as defined by Grossarth-Maticek, and cause of death (cancer or cardiovascular disease). These data convincingly demonstrate that the ancient belief in such a relationship is amply justified and can be securely established by modern methods of investigation.

It should be noted here that the personality type was established along three independent lines. Probands were shown verbal descriptions of the four personality types, and asked to indicate which of them was closest to their own particular pattern of behavior. A similar task was carried out by close friends or relatives who knew them well; this was of course done independently of the probands. Lastly, the interviewer also indicated his own view of the proband's position on the personality-type form. The three methods correlated quite highly together, suggesting a considerable degree of reliability to the ascertainment of probands' personality type; it was the self-rating that was used for establishing the results reported here.

The theories linking personality and cancer can usefully be extended to cover also duration of life after diagnosis, that is the ability of the organism and its immune system to combat the disease. There is considerable evidence for the existence of such a relation (Levy, 1985). Greer and colleagues (1979, 1985) found in a 10-year follow-up that women with breast cancer who were rated as showing a fighting spirit or who denied the significance of their illness had better outcomes than women who were rated as helpless or stoic. Rogentine and co-workers (1979) reported significantly greater relapse in melanoma patients showing a passive or stoic response style. Visintainer and Casey (1984) demonstrated a similar association between passivity and disease course in melanoma patients. Similar results are reported by Derogatis, Abelott, and Melisaratos (1979) in breast cancer patients, and Jensen (1984), also in breast cancer patients.

Levy (1985) reports a study linking personality and an immunological mediator (the natural killer cell, NK); NK activity was found to have prognostic significance. Patients who had higher levels of NK activity at the time of primary treatment had significantly fewer positive nodes. The crucial finding was that patients who were rated as "adjusted" by independent observers—who made no complaints and had no apparent psychological difficulties, and who responded with a listless, apathetic response style—tended to have significantly lower levels of NK activity than patients who appeared more disturbed. These latter patients tended to be more negatively reactive at the time of interview. "On the basis of these three factors—observer ratings of adjustment, perceived social support, and level of reported listlessness, we could account for 51% of the NK variance in these patients" (Levy, 1985, p. 167).

Animal studies have also given support to the hypothesis that "learned helplessness" is associated with cancer. Laudenslager, Ryan, Drugan, Higson, and Maier, (1983), Shavit, Gale, and Liebeskind, (1984), and Greenberg, Dyck, and Sandler (1984) suggest a causal relationship between acute behavioral helplessness in rats and mice, suppression of lymphocyte function, and faster tumor growth. This relationship seems to be modulated by endogenous opioids, because the experimental effects were reversed when an opioid antagonist was injected. These investigators also examined NK activity in the modulation of NK-specific tumors (YAC-1.3 and SL-5 NK-

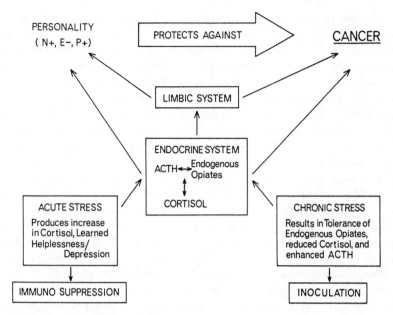

Figure 7.5 Diagrammatic form of causal analysis of the relationship between personality and cancer.

sensitive lymphoma cell lines). Shavit and colleagues also tested in vivo development and elimination of implanted mammary tumors in female rats. In most of this work the yoked "helpless" paradigm has been used in which the rat is given shocks that can be prevented by suitable action; the rat is yoked to another who receives identical shocks but is unable to prevent them. It is the uncontrollable shocks that produce stress leading to cancer, depleted brain norepinephrine levels, and depleted dopamine and serotonin levels in some brain areas, the extent and duration of the effects depending on age, strain of animal, and social housing conditions (Sklar & Anisman, 1981).

Causal hypotheses about the relationship between personality and disease have been suggested by Eysenck (1985b) and by Kanazir, Djordjevic-Markovic, and Grossarth-Maticek, (1984). Eysenck suggests that both personality and the immune system can be affected by features of the endocrine system, so that the apparent correlation between personality and cancer, say, is in fact mediated by ACTH, cortisol, the endogenous opiates, etc., which have been shown to affect both personality and the immune system. Thus for instance cortisol is known to be immunosuppressive and also to be related to stress responses of hopelessness and helplessness. Figure 7.5 shows in brief outline the essential features of this paradigm.

It is interesting to note that the data and their significance are little changed by correction for smoking habits. Indeed, one of the most interesting aspects of the Grossarth-Maticek studies is the fact that personality shows a much closer prospective relationship with cancer and cardiovascular disease than does smoking or drinking. Thus the current belief that mortality rates for cancer and cardiovascular disease would be considerably changed if there were changes in people's smoking habits does not seem well supported, and indeed attempts to get people to smoke less, change their cholesterol level by differential eating, and reduce blood pressure by suitable medical intervention have been found to have no effects on the actual death rate in treatment groups, as compared with control groups (Eysenck, 1985a).

In the above we have suggested a causal set of relationships, and this is important because the usual epidemiological type of study relies entirely on the discovery of correlations that may or may not have any kind of causal effect. The virtue of a causal hypothesis is that it leads to experiments that can support or disprove the hypothesis. What is the position here?

Let us first consider the recent work of Rodin (1980, 1986), which is very relevant to our hypothesis. Put briefly, Rodin studied old people in a home, subject to a variety of stresses, which according to the theory might lead to helplessness, depression, and death. Rodin introduced methods of coping with the stresses involved in various experimental groups, and compared their fate with that of members in control groups receiving either nothing or placebo instructions and treatments. The outcome was very clear-cut. Subjects who received appropriate instruction in coping behavior showed significantly higher nurses' ratings on such items as "happy; actively interested; sociable; self-initiating; vigorous." They also survived significantly longer than the nontreated subjects. Rodin also looked at cortisol levels, arguing that many deaths in elderly persons can be attributed to a general weakening of the immune system because corticosteroids display immunosuppressive properties (Gabrielson & Good, 1985). Indeed, as Rodin points out, there appears to be an inverse relationship between plasma corticosterone level and the capacity of the spleen to synthesize antibodies (Gisler, 1974). In healthy organisms there are usually homeostatic regulatory mechanisms effectively counteracting the suppressive properties of corticosteroids (Northey, 1965; Rose & Sabiston, 1971; Solomon, 1969). These homeostatic regulatory mechanisms may be less effective in the elderly (Timiras, 1972) so that stress without effective coping may have an even more debilitating effect on health in such people, through its effects on the pituitary-adrenal system.

As Rodin points out, ". . . this would occur because the magnitude of pituitary adrenocortical response to stress becomes greater with aging and environmental uncontrollability might exacerbate this condition" (p. 1995). To test this hypothesis, and the influence of effective coping on cortisol levels, she measured hypothalamo-pituitary adrenal activity by means of 24-hour urine samples. Three months prior to and 4 to 6 weeks after the intervention phase, urine was collected for free-cortisol (USC) measurements, the cortisol being measured in urine by radio immunoassay. Rodin noted first of all the initial high level of USC in the whole sample, followed by a significant reduction in the intervention groups, but not the no-treatment group. The self-instructional group, which showed a significant increase in coping responses after treatment as well as increased problem-solving activity and reduced stress from actual problems, showed high correlations between increased perceived control and increased problem-solving activity, with decreases in urinary-free cortisol levels of $r = .62$ and $.54$, respectively. This group also, unlike placebo-treatment groups, did not show a return to baseline after a 1-year follow-up as far as cortisol levels were concerned. Thus Rodin's work clearly supports the general hypothesis under investigation.

Turning now to cancer specifically, rather than survival in general, we have the important work of Grossarth-Maticek and co-workers (1983). He was concerned to supplement his prospective studies which, in spite of their superior methodology, could still only result in correlational findings, with a more experimental line of research that would provide direct evidence of the *causal* role of stress and coping mechanisms. In the first of these studies, women suffering from terminal cancer of the breast were given chemotherapy if they so desired. Of those who declined chemotherpy, half were treated by Grossarth-Maticek, using a type of behavior therapy he called "creative novation therapy." This is a kind of cognitive behavior therapy especially designed to relieve depression and hopelessness and encourage the expression of emotions. This method contains elements of Wolpe's method of desensitization, Beck's (1976) cognitive therapy of emotions disorders, and Lazarus and Folkman's (1984) method of teaching "coping strategies." In his own words, quoting from an unpublished manuscript:

> . . . creative novation therapy is a form of cognitive behaviour therapy, uniting the principles of learning underlying conventional behavioural techniques with certain cognitive principles. The therapy is designed to enable the patient to express needs that had previously been inhibited, and to engage in more satisfying social interactions. It is assummed that undesirable behaviour patterns are guided by cognitive-emotional programmes (values and assumptions) which can be modified. Through careful analysis the conflicting needs of the patient are identified. These are considered to be approach-avoidance conflicts, but are also similar to double-blind (e.g., "I love my husband who died years ago. I believed that I cannot live without him, therefore I wish to die to be reunited with him. But I also love to live and have good relations with my children."). The next therapeutic step is to define with the patient alternative behaviours and patterns of cognitive interpretation. No attempt is made to dismantle the structure of emotional needs (as in depth psychotherapy), but rather to bring resolution by substitution of new cognitive programmes (e.g., "I love my mother, but I have always thought I would betray her if I loved another woman. Now I realise that I am able to love both at the same time. Therefore I do not feel guilty anymore."). In addition, a programme of complete behavioural change is developed with the patient, and he or she is encouraged to work on these at home.

The design of the study thus gives us 4 groups, of 25 patients each. Some received both behavior therapy and chemotherapy, some neither, and some were given one but not the other. The dependent variable is length of survival in months. The group receiving neither type of therapy, with a mean survival time of 11.28 months, did worst, whereas the group receiving both therapies did best, with a mean survival time of 22.40 months. Those receiving only one or the other type of therapy showed a mean survival length of about 14.50 months, with the two types of therapy apparently equally successful in prolonging life. It is interesting that the combination of both is clearly synergistic, survival length being greater than the simple addition of the effects of the two types of therapy would suggest.

This synergistic effect may be illustrated by reference to the following figures. The mean survival time of all 100 patients was 15.7 months, with a standard deviation of 7.3 months, total survival time varying from 6 to 38 months. The relationship among behavior therapy, chemotherapy, and survival time was as follows: chemotherapy alone increased survival time by 2.80 months ($P < .001$), while behavior therapy alone increased survival by 3.64 months ($P < .001$). If the two effects were additive, one would expect a survival time of $11.28 + 2.80 + 3.64 = 17.72$ months for the groups with combined therapies. However, the mean survival time for the chemotherapy plus behavior therapy group was 22.40 months, exceeding the additive value by 4.68 ($P < .005$). This indicates that a positive interaction between chemotherapy and behavior therapy has taken place, and that they operate synergistically.

Additional patients, who had declined chemotherapy, were treated by orthodox behavior therapy or by psychoanalysis. Results for these methods were significantly worse than for creative novation therapy, and indeed dynamic psychotherapy did significantly worse than no therapy at all.

Is it possible to use creative novation therapy in a prophylactic manner for cancer, as Rodin used the teaching of coping behavior as a prophylactic treatment of stress in old age? In his Heidelberg prospective study, Grossarth-Maticek used 91 high cancer-prone subjects, 45 of whom were treated by means of creative novation therapy as a prophylactic measure, while the other 46 received no such therapy. Subjects were randomly allocated. Table 7.5 shows the results. It will be seen that of the patients who received behavior therapy, none died of cancer, whereas in the control group 12 died. Altogether 40 in the therapy group are still living, as compared with 25 in the control group. The difference is significant at the .0007 level.

Grossarth-Maticek carried out a similar study with 82 people who were prone to cardiovascular disease. Of the 43 people in the therapy group, 3 died of heart disease, whereas of the 39 control group, 14 died. Detailed results are given in Table 7.5. Again the difference between the two groups was very highly significant at the .009 level. These results obviously need replication, but they do suggest that there is a causal link between personality-related behavior patterns, their alteration by means of behavior therapy, and liability to contract various types of diseases.

Apart from the work of Rodin and Grossarth-Matick, there are other studies that show that it is possible to affect the development of physical di-

Table 7.5. Mortalities in the Two Therapy Intervention Studies: Heidelberg Stressed Sample

	Alive	Deceased from		
Risk: Cancer		Other Causes	Cancer	Total
Control group	25	9	12	46
Therapy group	40	5	0	45
Total	65	14	12	91

Significance: $\chi^2 = 0.0007$.

	Alive	Deceased from		
Risk: Infarct/Stroke		Other Causes	Infarct/stroke	Total
Control group	20	5	14	39
Therapy group	34	6	3	43
Total	54	11	17	82

Significance: $\chi^2 = 0.0090$.

sease by using behavior therapy methods to changed habitual behavior and emotional reactions. Thus Friedman and colleagues (1984) and Gill and colleagues (1985) have shown that groups of post-myocardial infarction patients who received group Type A behavior counseling, in comparison with control groups not receiving such counseling, showed significant cumulative cardiac recurrence rates significantly less than that observed in participants not receiving such counseling.

In the Friedman and colleagues studies (1984, 1986), 1,013 post-myocardial infarction patients were observed for 4.5 years to determine whether their Type A (coronary-prone) behavior could be altered and the effect such alteration might have on the subsequent cardiac morbidity and mortality rates of these individuals. Eight hundred sixty-two of these individuals were randomly assigned either to a control section of 270 participants who received group cardiac counseling or an experimental section of 592 participants who received both group cardiac counseling and Type-A behavioral counseling. The remaining 151 patients, serving as a comparison group, did not receive group counseling of any kind. Using the "Intention-to-Treat" principle, we observed markedly reduced Type A behavior at the end of 4.5 years in 35.1% of participants given cardiac and Type A behavior counseling compared with 9.8% of participants given only cardiac counseling. The cumulative 4.5-year cardiac recurrence rate was 12.9% in the 592 participants in the experimental group that received Type A counseling. This recurrence rate was significantly less ($P < 0.005$) than either the recurrence rate (21.2%) observed in the 270 participants in the control group or the recurrence rate (28.2%) in those of the comparison group not receiving any special treatment. After the first year, a significant difference in number of cardiac deaths between the experimental and control participants was observed during the remaining 3.5 years of the study. Overall, the results of this study demonstrate for the first time, within a controlled experimental design, that altering Type A behavior reduces cardiac morbidity and mortality in post-infarction patients.

It was also found (Gill et al., 1985) that subjects undergoing a profound reduction in the intensity of the Type A behavior pattern also exhibited a significantly lowered serum cholesterol value as the study continued, as compared with subjects who exhibited no change in their Type A behavior. Interesting as these data are, they are rather less impressive than those reported by Grossarth-Maticek, possibly because of the less satisfactory definition of the personality correlates involved in the "Type A" concept (Eysenck & Fulker, 1983).

Even more recently, Patel and co-workers (1985) allocated half of 192 coronary heart disease-prone men and women to an experimental group, the other half to a control group. Both groups were given health education leaflets containing advice to stop smoking, to reduce animal fats in their diets, and on the importance of reducing blood pressure. In addition, the treatment groups had group sessions of 1 hour a week for 8 weeks in which they were taught breathing excercises, relaxation and meditation, and about managing stress. After 4 years, more subjects in the control groups reported having had angina and treatment for hypertension. Incidence of ischemic heart disease and fatal myocardial infarction were significantly greater in the control groups.

Of special relevance to the application of the principles of behavior therapy is a study reported by Lovibond, Birrell, and Langeluddecke (1986). Seventy-five persons (57 male and 18 female) with a high risk of coronary heart disease (CHD) were randomly assigned in equal numbers to three 8-week behavioral treatment programs. All three treatments were designed to alter simultaneously a number of risk-elevating behavior patterns, in the expectation that change in any one behavior pattern would reinforce change in others. Weight, blood pressure, and aerobic fitness were regularly assessed in all subjects. Serum lipids were also measured, but less frequently. All three interventions produced significant beneficial changes in the major objective measures, and the changes were well maintained after 12 months. The most improved group exhibited the following mean changes: weight loss of 9.2kg, reductions in blood pressure of 12.9/8.8mm Hg, improvement in aerobic capacity of 33%, reduction in serum cholesterol of 0.45 mmol/liter, and deduction in current overall CHD risk of 41%. The effectiveness of the interventions was positively related to the degree to which the programs emphasized training in, and detailed application of, behavioral change principles.

Clearly the facts related in this brief account are of considerable interest in indicating a much closer relationship between psychology and medicine than might have been thought likely. In view of the fact that there have been several replications of the work linking personality and disease, it seems unlikely that this is no more than a statistical fallacy. The theories discussed, however, are obviously much more susceptible to change, and may be altogether along the wrong lines. At such an early stage it is difficult to be certain of one's claims, and much work clearly remains to be done to establish the truth or falsity of the theories in question. However, they are sufficiently precise to be tested, and deductions made from them are certain to be so tested in the near future. Particularly welcome, of course, is the conclusion that behavior therapy can be used prophylactically to prevent deaths from both cancer and cardiovascular disease, the two main killers at present. These findings in particular deserve replication and follow-up in many different countries in order to test the efficacy of the methods used, and to establish once and for all whether training in the methods of therapy used should be given to many medical people and psychologists employed in the health service. Altogether we seem to be at the beginning of a revolution in this field, and hopefully the results of this revolution will be socially desirable.

References

Beck, A.T. (1976). *Cognitive therapy and the emotional disorder*. New York: International Universities Press.

Derogatis, L.R., Abelott, M.D., & Melisaratos, N. (1979). Psychological coping mechanisms and survival time in metastatic breast cancer. *Journal of the American Medical Association, 242*, 1504–1509.

Eysenck, H.J. (1983). Stress, disease and personality: The "inoculation effect." In C.L. Cooper (Ed.), *Stress and research* (pp. 121–146). New York: John Wiley & Sons.

Eysenck, H.J. (1984). Personality, stress and lung cancer. In S. Rachman (Ed.), *Contributions to medical psychology*, Vol 3 (pp. 151–171). Oxford: Pergamon Press.

Eysenck, H.J. (1985a). Personality, cancer and cardiovascular disease: A causal analysis. *Personality and Individual Differences, 5*, 535–557.

Eysenck, H.J. (1985b). Smoking and health. In R. Tollison (Ed.), *Smoking and society* (pp. 17–88). Lexington, MA: D.C. Heath.

Eysenck, H.J. (1987a). Anxiety, "learned helplessness" and cancer—A causal theory. *Journal of Anxiety Disorders, 1*, 87–104.

Eysenck, H.J. (1987b). Personality as a predictor of cancer and cardiovascular disease and the application of behaviour therapy in prophylaxis. *European Journal of Psychiatry, 1*, 29–41.

Eysenck, H.J. (1988) (in press). The respective importance of personality, cigarette smoking and interaction effects for the genesis of cancer and coronary heart disease. *Personality and Individual Differences, 9* (in press).

Eysenck, H.J., & Fulker, D. (1983). The components of Type A behaviour and its genetic determinants. *Personality and Individual Differences, 5*, 499–505.

Friedman, M.D., Thoresen, C.E., Gill, J.J., Powell, L.H., Ulmer, D., Thompson, L., Price, V.A., Rabin, D.D., Brell, W.S., Dixon, T., Levy, R., & Bourg, E. (1984). Alterations of Type A behavior and reduction in cardiac recurrences in post-myocardial infarction patients. *American Heart Journal, 108*, 237–248.

Friedman, M., Thoresen, C., Gill, J., Ulmer, D., Powell, L.H., Price, V., Brown, B.,

Thompson, L., Rabin, D., Breall, W., Bourg, E., Levy, R., & Dixon, T. (1986). Alteration of Type A behaviour and its effect on cardiac recurrences in post-myocardial infarction patients: Summary results of the recurrent coronary prevention project. *American Heart Journal, 112,* 653–665.

Gabrielson, A.E., & Good, R.A. (1985). Chemical suppression of adaptive immunity. *Advances in Immunology, 110,* 503–514.

Gill, J.J., Price, V.A., Thoreson, C., Powell, L., Ulmer, D., Brown, B., Drews, F., & Friedman, M. (1985). Reduction in Type A behaviour in healthy middle-aged Australian military officers. *American Heart Journal, 110,* 503–514.

Gisler, R.H. (1974). Stress and the hormonal regulation of the immune response in mice. *Psychotherapy and Psychosomatics, 223,* 197.

Greenberg, A., Dyck, D., & Sandler, L. (1984). Opponent processes, neurohormones and natural resistance. In B. Fox & B. Newberry (Eds.), *Psychoneuroendocrine systems in cancer and immunity* (pp. 97–124). Toronto: Hogrefe.

Greer, S., Morris, T., & Pettingale, K. (1979). Psychological response to breast cancer: Effect and outcome. *Lancet, 2,* 785–787.

Greer, S., Morris, T., Pettingale, K., & Haylittle, J. (1985). Mental attitudes to cancer: An additional prognostic factor. *Lancet, 1,* 750.

Grossarth-Maticek, R. (1980). Synergic effects of cigarette smoking, systonic blood pressure, and psychosocial risk factors for lung cancer, cardiac infarct and apoplexi cerebri. *Psychotherapy and Psychosomatics, 34,* 267–272.

Grossarth-Maticek, R., Eysenck, H.J., & Vetter, H. (1987). (in press). Personality type, cancer and coronary heart disease. *Personality and Individual Differences.*

Grossarth-Maticek, R., Eysenck, H.J., Vetter, H., & Frentzel-Beyme, R. (1986). The Heidelberg prospective intervention study. Paper presented at the First International Symposium on Primary Prevention and Cancer, Antwerp, Belgium, March 1922.

Grossarth-Maticek, R., Kanazir, D.T., Schmidt, P., & Vetter, H. (1982). Psychosomatic factors in the process of cancerogenesis. *Psychotherapy and Psychosomatics, 28,* 284–302.

Grossarth-Maticek, R., Kanazir, D.T., Schmidt, P., Vetter, H., & Jankovic, M. (1983). Psychosomatic factors in the process of cancerogenesis. *Psychotherapy and Psychosomatics, 39,* 94–105.

Jensen, G. (1984). Psychobiological factors in the prognosis and treatment of neoplastic disorder. Unpublished doctoral dissertation, Department of Psychology, Yale University, New Haven, CT. Quoted in Levy, 1985.

Kanazir, D., Djordjevic-Markovic, R., & Grossarth-Maticek, R. (1984). Psychosocial factors, emotional stress, steroid hormones and carcinogenesis: Molecular aspects, facts and speculations. In Y.A. Ouchinnikov (Ed.), *Progress in biorganic chemistry and molecular biology* (pp. 509–530). Amsterdam: Elsevier Science Publishers.

Kissen, D.M., & Eysenck, H.J. (1962). Personality in male lung cancer patients. *J Psychosomatic Research, 6,* 123–137.

Laudenslager, M.L., Ryan, S.M., Drugan, R.C., Higson, R.L., & Maier, S.F. (1983). Coping and immunosupression. Inescapable but not escapable shock suppresses lymphocyte proliferation. *Science, 221,* 568–570.

Lazarus, R.S., & Folkman, S. (1984). *Stress, appraisal and coping.* New York: Springer.

Levy, S. (1985). *Behaviour and cancer.* London: Jossey-Bass Publishers.

Lovibond, S.H., Birrell, P., & Langeluddecke, P. (1986). Changing coronary heart disease risk-factor status: The effects of three behavioural programs. *Journal of Behavioural Medicine, 9,* 415–437.

Northey, W.T. (1965). Studies on the interrelationship of cold environment, immunity and resistance to infection. 1. Qualitative and quantitative studies on the immune response. *Journal of Immunology, 94,* 649.

Patel, C., Mammot, M.G., Terry, D.J., Carruthers, M., Hunt, B., & Patel, M. (1985). Trial of relaxation in reducing coronary risks: A four-year follow-up. *British Medical Journal, 290,* 1103–1106.

Rodin, J. (1980). Managing the stress of aging: The role of control and coping. In S. Levine, & H. Ursin, (Eds.), *Coping and health* (pp. 193–204). New York: Plenum Press.

Rodin, J. (1986). Health, control and aging. In M.M. Baltes & P.B. Baltes (Eds.), *Aging and the psychology of control* (pp. 113–129). Hillsdale, NJ: Plenum Press.

Rogentine, N., Daniel P., Fox, B., Docherty, J.P., Rosenblatt, J., Boyd, S., & Bunney, W. (1979). Psychological factors in the prognosis of malignant melanoma: A prospective study. *Psychosomatic Medicine, 41,* 647–655.

Rose, J.E.M. St., & Sabiston, B.H. (1971). Effects of cold exposure on the immunologic response of rabbits to human serum albumin. *Journal of Immunology, 107,* 339.

Schmidt, P. (1984). Autoritarismus, Entfremdung und psychosomatische Krebsforschung: Explikation der drei Forschungs—programme durch eine allgemeine Theorie und empirische Tests mittels strukturvergleichung [Authoritarianism, alienation and psychosomatic study of cancer: Explication of three programs of investigation—in terms of general theory and empirical tests using the comparison of structures.] Unpublished doctoral thesis, University of Giessen, Giessen, West Germany.

Shavit, J., Gale, R.P., & Liebeskind, J.C. (1984). Opioid peptides mediate the suppressive effect of stress in natural killer cell cytotoxicity. *Science, 273,* 188–190.

Sklar, L., & Anisman, H. (1981). Stress and cancer. *Psychological Bulletin, 89,* 309–406.

Solomon, G.F. (1969). Stress and antibody response in rats. *Internat Archives of Illness, 9,* 35, 97.

Timiras, P.S. (1972). *Developmental physiology and aging.* New York: Macmillan.

Visintainer, M.A., & Casey, R. (1984). Adjustment and outcome in melanoma patients. Paper presented at meeting of the American Psychological Association, Toronto. Quoted by Levy, 1985.

8

Temperamental Dimensions as Co-Determinants of Resistance to Stress

Jan Strelau

This final chapter by Strelau provides a fitting conceptual framework, the Regulative Theory of Temperament (RTT), in which to consider the reviews, data, and theory presented in the previous seven chapters. As have others, Strelau views stress as resulting from an interaction between the environment and the organism—thus if stress were solely an external factor, the need to understand differences among organisms would not be necessary. As this is not the case, the study of individual differences becomes the *sine qua non* for understanding stress. He decries the relative lack of attention that this aspect of stress has generated. If, as Strelau and others believe, stress is a state caused by a lack of equilibrium between environmental demands and the ability to cope, again the need to consider individual differences is underscored. In the context of the RTT approach, the major determinant of an organism's response to stress is *reactivity*, the individual's typical and stable intensity of response to a stimulus. Reactivity is viewed as the most important individual difference construct in understanding stress reactions. In the concluding portions of his chapter Strelau marshals an impressive array of evidence to substantiate this claim, covering such topics as performance, psychophysiology, and coping. The reactivity approach to studying the stress response may provide a perspective for many scientists that opens broad avenues of new thinking on an old issue.

—EDITOR

Hundreds, if not thousands of books and papers have been published with the aim of presenting different aspects of psychological stress. Studies in this area pay little attention to the significance of individual differences in stress. This is especially true as regards the first stage of research in this area.

The *idiosyncratic* approach to the study of different aspects of stress—a good starting point to focus in on individual differences—has been systematically developed by Lazarus (1966; Opton & Lazarus, 1967). For several years it has been accepted by many psychologists involved in stress research (e.g., Appley & Trumbull, 1967; Chan, 1977; Krohne & Rogner, 1982; Lacey, 1967; Magnusson, 1982; McGrath 1970b; Schulz & Schönpflug, 1982).

The significance of individual differences in approaching stress differs depending on the understanding of the *nature* of stress. Without going into detail, one should agree with McGrath (1970a) who argues that there was/ is almost no place for individual differences if stress would be regarded as an *external factor*, as a stress-inducing situation (e.g., Weick, 1970). Even if one regards stress as the *response* (reaction) to given stressors, which is in line with Selye's understanding of stress (1956, 1975), the place for individual differences is limited.

The importance of individual differences in research on stress has become clear since stress began to be regarded as a *state* that is the outcome of *interaction* between the stress-inducing environment (stressor) and the individual, including his or her physical, as well as psychological characteristics (Magnusson, 1982; McGrath, 1970a).

> What becomes a stressor is not determined solely by the nature of the situation or by the individual and his disposition. A stress reaction in an individual is the joint effect of his psychic and somatic dispositions *and* the stress provoking quality of situational conditions, the stressors (Magnusson, 1982, p. 234).

Most psychologists involved in stress research undertaken at the interactional level agree with Lazarus (1966) that *appraisal of the perceived situation* should be treated as an important variable in determining psychological stress, the latter being regarded as *threat* (see also Appley & Trumbull, 1967; Magnusson, 1982; McGrath, 1982). The process of appraisal that takes place in the individual is always a *subjective* one, and this means, among other things, that it runs differently in different people. If we take this understanding of stress as a point of departure, then the conclusion must be that the individual differences approach should be considered as one of the most important paradigms in the study of stress. For "individual differences, styles, patterns of response, and prepotent tendencies appear to be the rule rather than the exception in studies of psychological stress" (Appley & Trumbull, 1967, p. 4).

Sources of Individual Differences in Studying Stress

The sources of individual differences that should be taken into account when studying stress are innumerable. Therefore to build a commonly accepted taxonomy in order to review them systematically is almost impossible. Recently (Strelau, in press), I presented a preliminary list of some of those factors that might be regarded as sources of individual differences within the different aspects of studying stress, including the perception of stress-inducing situations, the reactions to stress, as well as coping with stress. Without detailing the separate sources (which can be found elsewhere, e.g., Strelau [in press]), I will limit myself to their presentation and to some general remarks.

Individual Differences in Appraising Whether the Same Objective Situation is Threatening

What is regarded as threatening for one individual may be treated as less threatening, or not at all threatening for another (Lazarus, 1966; McGrath, 1970b). The differences in perceiving given situations as being threatening may also be considered within one individual only. What he or she perceives as a source of threat at a given moment may not be appraised as threatening in another period of life, or in another place. Thus, inter- as well as intra-individual differences exist in objectively appraising the same situation as being a stressor. The list of sources for these differences includes at least the following:

1. the individual's life history;
2. the developmental- and individual-specific cognitive map (network);
3. experience with stress-inducing situations;
4. system of motivation and the accepted system of values;
5. the structure and sensitivity of the receptor; and
6. the actual (physical and psychic) state of the individual.

Individual Differences in Reactions to Stressors

The variety of reactions to a stressor—independent of whether they will be regarded as consequences of stress, as stress itself, or as indicators of the state of stress—depends not only on the kind of stress-inducing situations, but also upon the individual himself, and here again exist strongly expressed inter- as well as intra-individual differences. These may be considered, among other things, from the following points of view:

1. preferences of the kind (level) of activity being regarded as a response to stress;
2. individual differences in behavior;
3. individual differences in psychic states; and
4. individual differences in physiological reactions.

Individual Differences in Coping with Stress

The state of stress in itself may occur or not. The stressors may be perceived as more or less threatening, depending on the degree to which the individual is able to cope with stress, or what repertoire of coping mechanisms is activated during stress. The importance of coping with stress in human behavior has been described by Lazarus (1966, 1967; Monat & Lazarus, 1985), who distinguishes two main coping mechanisms with stress—direct actions and defense mechanisms. Schulz and Schönpflug (1982) have regarded the inadequate coping behavior as the main condition for the occurrence of stress. It is not possible here to detail the nature of coping mechanisms for stress and the role they play in human behavior, which have been discussed by many authors (e.g., Cox, 1978; Fenz, 1975; Lazarus, 1966, 1967; Meichenbaum, 1977; Monat & Lazarus, 1985). However, it should be mentioned that the individual-differences approach in studying these mechanisms may help in their proper understanding. Individual differences in coping with stress may reveal themselves in different ways, some of them are mentioned below:

1. direct actions versus defense mechanisms—individual differences in preferences;
2. individual differences in defense mechanisms of coping with stress;
3. individual differences in direct actions aimed at coping with stress;
4. individual differences in capacities and acquired skills in coping with stress; and
5. individual differences in the repertoire of strategies aimed at coping with stress.

Personality Dimensions as Sources of Individual Differences in Stress

In the individual differences approach to studies on stress, a special place should be given to personality and temperament traits. As has been stressed by Lazarus ". . . the objective stimulus situation is appraised on the basis of its characteristics as well as traits of personality. . . ." (1967, p. 164). The impact of personality dimensions in co-determining stress and the resistance to stress differs according to the type of situation regarded as being stress-inducing, the individual himself, and also on the specificity of his personality trait being taken into account (see Chan, 1977; Cox, 1978).

Personality Traits with Limited Contribution in Co-Determining Tolerance to Stress

One may assume that in many stress-inducing situations some personality dimensions may not be at all important in determining the state of stress, or their importance is low and/or limited in scope. For example, a high position on the dimension of objectivity probably does not influence the individual's reactions and behavior when he is attacked by an aggressive and dangerous dog. If we take another personality dimension into account, for example, level of aspiration, then it might be assumed that for individuals with a high

level of aspiration, an examination situation, or a situation of competition
will be perceived as more threatening than for individuals with a low level
of aspiration. This personality dimension may at the same time have no
influence on perceiving other situations as being threatening. Dozens of
personality traits (dimensions) may be mentioned here as examples illus-
trating that their impact in determining individual differences in stress is
very selective and limited.

It is highly probable that personality dimensions, the variance of which is
mainly determined by social factors, have a strongly expressed situation-
specific and reaction-specific influence (see Endler & Magnusson, 1976; Mischel, 1969) on molding individual differences in stress. The reason is that
they are determined by social-specific interactions and they develop under
the individual's specific experience. One can assume that the influence of
personality factors determined mainly by social learning is especially evident
when individual differences in coping with stress are considered (e.g., Kobasa, 1979). For example, whether an individual prefers direct actions or involves defense mechanisms in coping with stress depends largely on whether
approach-specific or avoidance-specific personality dimensions have been
developed in ontogenesis. The system of reinforcement used by parents and
other important persons in case of successful and/or unsuccessful behavior in
stress-inducing situations leads to individual differences in *styles* of coping
with stress.

Many personality dimensions might be mentioned here as examples of
traits that may co-determine to a high degree whether or not a situation is
appraised as being threatening. They may also co-determine the type of reaction in which the state of stress might be expressed, as well as the way in
which the individual copes with stress. It is assumed here that of special
significance are the biologically determined personality dimensions based on
the concept of activation (see Strelau & Eysenck, 1987). For reasons presented elsewhere (see Strelau, 1982, 1987a) I prefer to consider them under
the label *temperament*.

The Role of Temperamental Traits in Determining Stress

In discussing the relation between stress and temperamental traits, I refer to
the understanding of stress as a state caused by the lack of equilibrium (imbalance) between environmental demands and the individual's capability
to cope with them (see Laux & Vossell, 1982; McGrath, 1970a; Schulz &
Schönpflug, 1982), paying special attention to the energetic aspect of the
relationship: environment–individual.

The Concept of Stress Considered from the Energetic Point of View

In spite of limiting the cognitive appraisal of the demand-capability imbalance almost to threat, regarded as the synonym of *psychological stress*
(Lazarus, 1966; McGrath, 1970a, 1982), let me take as a starting point the

understanding of stress proposed by Selye (1956; see also 1982). He considers the nonspecificity of demands (stressors) and the nonspecific response to these demands (stress) as the essence of his theory. As Selye writes: "*It is immaterial whether the agent or situation we face is pleasant or unpleasant*; all that counts is the intensity of the demand for readjustment or adaptation" (1975, p. 15).

Thus the intensity of demands (stimuli) is the crucial factor (stressor) causing stress. The stress response will be stronger the more extreme (on both directions on the intensity dimensions of demands) the stimuli are. As Selye has said, "Deprivation of stimuli and excessive stimulation are both accompanied by an increase in stress, sometimes to the point of distress" (1975, p. 21).

Selye regards his concept of stress as a response-based being, in essence a biological phenomenon, although produced by environmental factors. It is often described as *systemic stress* (see Appley & Trumbull, 1967). If we take into account, however, that the intensity of agents causing stress depends not only on the agents themselves, but above all on the individual's cognitive appraisal of these agents and on his or her *tolerability* (Lazarus, 1966) or *vulnerability* (Appley & Trumbull, 1967) to stressors—in which individuals differ—then we have to use a psychological concept of stress based on an interactional paradigm. The essence of the concept of stress presented here consists in paying attention to the *intensity of stimulation* and to the *capability of the individual to cope with stimuli of extreme value*—both deprivation as well as strong stimuli. The intensity of stimulation is determined by the stimuli themselves, by the physiological process of individual-specific stimulus intensity modulation, as well as by the individual's cognitive appraisal.

The state of stress is caused by the imbalance between the individual's capacity (determined by external and internal conditions) to respond to stimuli of different intensities and the stimulation value of the situation; the stimulative value is determined by objectively existing features (intensity, complexity, etc.) as well as by the subjective processes.

The intensity of stimulation (stressor) has been regarded by Selye (1956, 1975) as a nonspecific agent causing stress. Also, authors discussing the concept of psychological stress consider the intensity of stimulation as a source of stress (see Lundberg, 1982; McGrath, 1970c; Weick, 1970), which allows us to relate the concept of stress to the level of arousal (activation). Taking as a point of departure the Yerkes-Dodson law and Hebb's (1955) concept of arousal, one may conclude that situations or stimuli above and below the individual's need for stimulation evoke a state of discomfort, the state of stress, which leads to changes in physiological, psychological, and behavioral reactions as well as in the level of performance (see Lundberg, 1982).

Arousal-Oriented Temperament Dimensions as Co-Determinants of Stress

If we take as a starting point the conclusion following from the former discussion, which says that the intensity of agents causing stress depends not only on the agents themselves but also on the individual-specific stimulation processing (modulation of physiological intensity of stimuli and cognitive appraisal) and on the individual's tolerability or—the opposite—vulnerability to stressors; then it becomes clear that personality or temperament dimensions that refer to the level of arousal are of special significance in determining individual differences in stress.

Under high levels of arousal the tolerability to stressors of high intensity is lowered, caused by the process of augmentation of acting stimuli. Under low levels of arousal there occurs a decrease in tolerability to stimuli of low stimulative value (e.g., deprivation), this being the result of suppression processes regarding the value of already low stimulation.

Arousal-oriented temperament dimensions are based on the assumption that there exist more or less stable individual differences in the level of arousal. Some individuals are permanently rather highly aroused whereas others have a chronically low level of arousal. To underline the fact that there exist relatively stable individual differences in the level of arousal, Gray (1964) introduced the concept of *arousability*. In individuals characterized by high arousability, stimuli of given intensity (Sn) develop a high level of arousal (An + x); whereas in individuals having low arousability, the level of arousal to the same stimuli is lower (An − x). This might be expressed as follows:

$$Sn \rightarrow An + x = \text{high arousability}$$
$$Sn \rightarrow An - x = \text{low arousability}$$

There are several dimensions of personality/temperament that refer to the concepts of arousal and arousability. The main differences between them, from the energetic point of view, consists in the fact that they concentrate on different anatomical and physiological mechanisms underlying arousal, as well as on different aspects of behavior in which arousal is expressed. Such dimensions include extraversion-introversion, sensation seeking, anxiety, neuroticism, augmenting-reducing, strength of the nervous system, and reactivity (see Strelau, 1985, 1987b; Strelau & Eysenck, 1987).

To illustrate the influence of arousal-oriented personality or temperamental traits on determining individual differences in stress, let me take the Eysenckian extraversion-introversion dimension as an example. As is already well known, the reticulo-cortical arousal loop has been regarded by Eysenck (1967, 1970) as the physiological mechanism of extraversion-introversion. Extraverts should be characterized as having a generally lower level of arousal as compared with introverts for whom a high level of arousal is rather typical. It can be learned from the literature devoted to stress (e.g., Lazarus, 1966; Lundberg, 1982; Selye, 1975) that there is a close relationship between the individual's level of arousal, the stimulative value of the threatening situation, and the state of stress.

Extraversion-introversion should be regarded as an important factor in co-determining whether or not a situation is appraised as being threatening. Referring to Wundt (1874), Eysenck looks at the fact that extraversion-introversion co-determines whether a stimulation of given intensity should be regarded as evoking a positive hedonic tone or a negative hedonic tone (Eysenck, 1981a). By taking Selye's position we could say that both extremes (high positive and high negative hedonic tones) have much in common with stress, whereas regarding stress as a state evoked by threatening situations, the negative hedonic tone may be considered as synonymous with stress. Where introverts are concerned, stimuli of lower intensity evoke a negative hedonic tone (the state of stress) as compared with extraverts, and the range of stimuli that evoke this state will be broader where introverts are concerned.

A great deal of evidence has been collected by Eysenck (1981b) and his students, which shows that a specific interrelation exists between level of performance and the stimulative value of situations, depending on whether we are dealing with extraverts or introverts. From those regularities it should be clear that as far as the state of stress in relation to level of performance is considered—and this is one of the most common approaches in stress research (e.g., Broverman, Klaiber, Vogel, & Kobayashi, 1974; Lundberg, 1982; McGrath, 1970a)—we have to regard extraversion-introversion as one of the individual's most important traits taking part in the interplay between the stimulative value of the situation perceived as being threatening, and in the individual's level of performance (see Brebner, in press; Eysenck, 1981b; Morris, 1979; Schalling, 1976; Schönpflug, 1982; Schulz & Schönpflug, 1982).

It would require a longer chapter than this to draw the whole picture for an understanding of the interrelationships between extraversion-introversion and stress. One of the main purposes here is to indicate the place of reactivity, regarded as a temperament dimension, in co-determining the resistance to stress.

Reactivity as a Co-Determinant of Resistance to Stress

Theoretical Background

In our concept of temperament, known as the Regulative Theory of Temperament (RTT) (see Strelau, 1983a, 1983b, 1986), special attention is paid to traits that refer to the energetic aspects of behavior, reactivity and activity. To show the interrelationships between stress and reactivity, the latter concept is briefly described.

The Concept of Reactivity

According to the RTT reactivity is conceived as a property due to which an individual is marked by a relatively stable and typical intensity of response to stimuli. When it comes to measurement, one may say that the intensity or the magnitude of individual response is estimated by comparing it with the

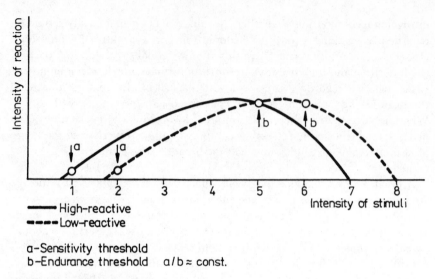

Figure 8.1. Model of intensity (magnitude) of reactions in high- and low-reactive individuals (taken from Strelau, 1983a).

intensity of reactions of other persons to the same stimulus. We make an assumption here that the administered stimulus has a similar value for each person or else is neutral. Reactivity co-determines the *sensitivity* as measured by sensory threshold and the organism's *endurance* (capacity to work), manifested in reaction to strong or prolonged stimulation. This is similar to the interpretation of Pavlov's concept of the nervous system strength as the capacity for adequate response to a high intensity stimuli, a long term stimulus, or one that occurs repeatedly (Pavlov, 1951–1952). As studies on nervous system strength carried out by Soviet psychologists (Nebylitsyn, 1972) indicate, there is a relatively stable dependency between sensitivity and endurance.

The weaker the stimulus that elicits a perceptible response (and thus a higher sensitivity) and the weaker the stimulus that starts to lower efficiency (a lower capacity), the higher the reactivity of an individual, and conversely, a low-reactive person is marked by low sensitivity and high endurance (see Figure 8.1).

Without delving into details of the physiological mechanism of reactivity, we can say that in high-reactive individuals this mechanism reinforces stimulation. Certain stimuli received from outside as well as inside the organism evoke stronger responses in these persons in comparison with weakly reactive individuals. Speaking in line with my co-worker, Matysiak (1980), high-reactive individuals are marked by a high stimulation processing coefficient (SPC). Low-reactive individuals on the other hand possess a physiological mechanism for suppressing stimulation, which means that stimuli of a definite strength elicit in them a lesser reaction than in more reactive individuals. In other words, weakly reactive individuals have a low SPC. Coefficient values denoting the physiological mechanism of energetic stimulation processing are most likely distributed according to Gauss's curve. Therefore we speak of high versus low SPC in order to emphasize the differences appearing in this respect between individuals (groups).

High-reactive individuals, in whom the physiological mechanism is marked by a high SPC, have a low need for stimulation to attain optimal level of activation, the latter being regarded here as a *standard of stimulus intensity regulation* (see Eliasz, 1985; Strelau, 1983a). On the other hand, low-reactive individuals, having a low SPC provide themselves with a larger number of stimuli in order to maintain the optimal level of activation and thus they show a high need for stimulation. Therefore, highly reactive individuals avoid stimulations and activities that bring along strong stimulation, whereas low-reactive persons undertake activities and seek out situations that possess a high stimulating quality. In consequence, weakly reactive individuals are generally more active and highly reactive ones show lowered activity.

Turning back to the concept of arousability (Gray, 1964), we can say that high-reactive individuals, because of their high SPC and thus high sensitivity, are characterized by a high level of arousability. Low-reactive individuals for whom a low SPC and thus low sensitivity is typical, have a low level of arousability.

The Interrelations Between Stress and Reactivity

Because reactivity refers mainly to the energetic characteristics of behavior, it seems reasonable to seek interrelationships between this temperamental feature and stress, regarding the stress from also the energetic perspective. As mentioned above, the essence of such an understanding of the phenomenon of stress consists of the lack of equilibrium between the stimulative value of demands and the capability of the individual to cope with these demands.

In high-reactive individuals, whose physiological mechanism intensifies stimulation (with low sensory sensitivity threshold and low endurance), a given situation has higher stimulative value in comparison with low-reactive individuals. Hence it appears that situations of high-stimulative value that do not evoke the state of stress in low-reactive individuals (who have a high need for stimulation) evoke this state in high-reactive individuals (who have a low need for stimulation). The opposite may be said to be true in situations characterized by a low stimulative value. A situation of deprivation that may evoke a state of discomfort (stress) in low-reactive individuals may be perceived as adequate for individuals with a high level of reactivity, because in this case the same situation has a higher stimulative value.

The state of stress considered here as the lack of equilibrium between the demands—which include the stimulative value of situations as well as of the tasks the individual is confronted with, and his capability to cope with stress, limited here to the individual's level of reactivity—may express itself in different ways.

When demands are of high stimulative value, the state of stress occurs first of all in high reactives; this is expressed in a decrease of performance as compared with results obtained in normal situations and/or in comparison with the level of performance of low reactives under high stimulative demands.

When the lack of equilibrium between demands and the individual's tolerability is caused by the extremely low stimulative value of demands (e.g., deprivation), the level of performance is higher in highly reactive individuals as compared with the low reactives, thus suggesting that this situation evokes a state of stress in the low reactives.

In the stress literature, it is acknowledged that the maintenance of high and constant performance under stress-inducing stimulation (overload or underload) may lead to several psychophysiological changes or side-effects that may be classified as psychophysiological cost (e.g., Glass & Singer, 1972; Lundberg & Frankenhaeuser, 1978). The coronary-prone Type A (Friedman & Rosenman, 1974) is an extreme example of the price an individual pays in order to maintain a given performance level. These psychophysiological changes will be expressed less in individuals resistant to stress than in nonresistant individuals. Under highly stimulative demands high-reactive individuals pay higher costs as compared with low-reactive ones in order to solve the task; these costs are regarded as an indicator of the state of stress (see Klonowicz, 1974, 1985; Strelau, 1983a).

In order to avoid the state of stress, high- and low-reactive individuals use different strategies and styles to cope with stressors. In low-reactive individuals the lack of equilibrium between the stimulative value of demands and their capability to cope with them (the state of stress) is caused mainly by the fact that these demands are *under* their capability. Thus they tend to develop in ontogenesis such activities that are of high stimulative value. This may be expressed, for example, in a tendency to undertake risky behaviors or in developing a style of action called the straightforward style of action.

In highly reactive individuals the lack of equilibrium between the stimulative value of demands and the individual's capacity to cope with them is determined first of all by their low tolerability to demands of high stimulative value. Thus in order to avoid the state of stress, they develop such behavior strategies as risk-avoiding activities or so-called adjunctive style of action. As far as risk-taking and risk-avoiding strategies of behavior are concerned we understand more or less to what kind of behavior they refer to. The styles of action mentioned here need explanation, however.

The style of action, understood as the typical manner in which an action is performed by the individual, develops under environmental influences on the basis of the temperamental endowment (especially reactivity and mobility of behavior). It is considered in the RTT (see Strelau, 1983a) as one of the *regulators of stimulation need*. The style of action refers to the functional aspect of activity. According to Tomaszewski (1978), taking into consideration the role that the separate components of activity play, all activities may be divided into basic or executive and auxiliary activities.

Those activities that lead directly to the attainment of a certain goal should be regarded as *basic*. The function of *auxiliary activities* consists of organizing conditions for the performance of primary activities. Auxiliary activities may be divided into orienting, preparatory, corrective, controlling, and protective activities (Tomaszewski, 1978). They raise the probability of attaining the goal of the performed action. In other words, auxiliary actions lower the risk of failure in task performance under stressors. Considering the relation between auxiliary and basic actions from the point of view of intensity of stimulation means that auxiliary actions, by safeguarding, facilitating, or simplifying the basic ones, lower the stimulative value of activity or the situation in which the activity is performed. From this it follows that high-reactive individuals will undertake more auxiliary actions to decrease the stimulative value of the performed activity (or situation in which activity is performed) as compared with low-reactive individuals.

One may assume (see Strelau, 1983a) that in high-reactive individuals auxiliary actions (AA) will dominate over basic ones (BA), thus the *adjunctive style of action* is typical for them. In low-reactive individuals there will be more of an equilibrium between both types of action or even a predominance of executive actions, this being typical for the *straightforward style of action*. This regularity may be expressed as follows:

High-reactives: BA < AA (adjunctive style)
Low-reactives: BA ⩾ AA (straightforward style)

Taking recourse to auxiliary actions, high-reactive persons may avoid stressors that might considerably lower their efficiency or productivity. Thus high-reactive persons may attain the same level of effect in their activity as do low-reactive persons.

Empirical Evidence

The hypotheses regarding the interrelations between the reactivity trait and resistance to stress, and the ways of coping with stress in high-reactive individuals have been examined in our laboratory, as well as by other investigators in many experiments (e.g., Danilova, 1985; Eliasz, 1981, 1985; Klonowicz, 1974, 1984, 1985; Mündelein, 1982; Przymusiński & Strelau, 1986; Strelau, 1983a, 1986; Żmudzki, 1986). It is impossible here to refer to all of them, thus in order to exemplify the regularities found in most of the studies related to the interrelationships between reactivity and stress I will limit this presentation to selected data.

Reactivity and Level of Performance Under Stressors

As mentioned before, it is expected that under demands of highly stimulative value the level of performance in high- and low-reactive individuals will be different in favor of the low reactives. Some of the data supporting this regularity have been presented elsewhere (e.g., Strelau, 1983a).

Probably one of the most spectacular situations in which this regularity occurs is sports activity. Competitions, especially those that, for different reasons are important for the participating contestant, are of high stimulative value. This is caused, among other things, by such factors as social appraisal, shame when losing, a chance for winning, and probability of receiving a prize.

Żmudzki (1986), in a study conducted on 75 weight lifters representing the Polish national team (average age 23.2 years), was able to show that the efficiency of performance during starts in national and international competitions, regarded as highly stressful situations, was different depending on the level of reactivity. Highly reactive weight lifters performed significantly lower (t = 2.768, $p < .01$) as compared with low-reactive individuals (see Figure 8.2).

Level of reactivity was estimated on the basis of the Strelau Temperament Inventory (STI). Taking as the criterion the quartile deviation, the author

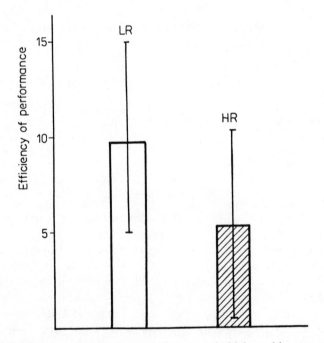

Figure 8.2. Efficiency of performance during starts in high- and low-reactive weight lifters (adapted from Zmudzki, 1986).

separated among the 75 subjects 19 low-reactive (LR) and 18 high-reactive (HR) individuals. The efficiency of performance during 10 different national and international competitions was estimated by means of a 7-point scale that included such items as absolute level of performance (of the snatch and jerk), the result obtained in comparison with the weight lifter's life record, with his efficiency during training, and with his constitutionally determined capacity.

It has to be stressed here that this study is of special interest because the efficiency of performance has been measured in natural situations (real competitions) and the result expressed here in a single number is an outcome of studies conducted in 10 different situations, all of them being of the same kind and characterized as highly demanding.

In several of our studies we concentrated on the influence of the interaction between the stimulative value of the situation and reactivity on the level of performance. For example, Klonowicz (1984, 1987) conducted an experiment, the aim of which was, among other things, to study the influence of the interaction between the level of reactivity, as measured by STI, and the stimulative value of situation on the efficiency of performance during one hour of work consisting of proofreading. As one of the indicators of efficiency of performance, the proportion of errors index (i.e., the misprints left uncorrected) has been used. Three situations differing in stimulation were arranged: quiet (40–46 dB), white noise (approximately 82 dB), and street noise (about 82 dB). It was assumed that street noise, because of its strong distractive influence on the performance of mental tasks, has a stronger stimulative value as compared with white noise. The subjects under study were 19 to 20-year-old female students, 39 HR and 39 LR individuals selected from a larger preliminary group by means of the quartile deviation. Some of the results of this study are displayed in Figure 8.3.

As can be seen, the effect of stimulation by reactivity interaction is evident and statistically significant ($F/2.72/ = 14.500, p < .001$). Taking into account the simple effects, Klonowicz stated that low reactives improved their performance as the stimulation load increased, whereas in high reactives the opposite occurred.

Moreover, these data show that low reactives apparently benefit from the fact that additional stimulation was imposed over a monotonous task; high reactives were adversely affected by both the intensity of stimulation and its nature: Variable stimulation (street noise) produced more deficits in performance than invariant (white noise) stimulation ($t = 2.28, p < .02$) (Klonowicz, 1987, pp. 187–188).

If we consider the performance of a monotonous task (proofreading) under quiet conditions as an underloaded stimulation (thus a type of stressor) for LR individuals and the same performance under street noise as an overloaded stimulation (i.e., stressor) for HR individuals, then the regularities stated in this experiment become understandable.

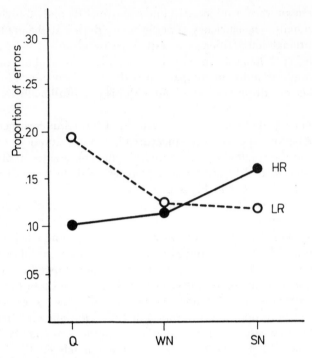

Figure 8.3. Proportion of errors as a function of interaction of reactivity × stimulation (taken from Klonowicz, 1985).

Reactivity and Psychophysiological Costs of Efficient Performance Under Stress

As mentioned before, it is expected that in highly stimulative situations the psychophysiological costs should be more pronounced in high-reactive individuals, whereas the reverse should occur when low stimulation (monotony or deprivation) is experienced. In this case the psychophysiological costs should be higher in low-reactive individuals. In our laboratory, Klonowicz (1974, 1984, 1985) has conducted several studies to investigate the relation between level of reactivity, stimulative value of a situation, and the psychophysiological costs paid by the individual during task performance. Her first experiment in this area, described in the following paragraph, seems to be especially illustrative (see Klonowicz, 1974).

Two groups of subjects radically differing in reactivity and exposed to situations of different stimulation load were studied. The less stimulating condition involved the application of Mackworth's vigilance test (auditory version), in which subjects are asked to respond by pressing a key to stimuli of double duration as opposed to neutral ones. All in all, 24 such stimuli were presented at irregular intervals (ranging from 30 seconds to 10 minutes). The neutral stimuli were presented at regular intervals for one hour. The more stimulating condition required subjects to work as efficiently as possible on a modified version of Krapelin's arithmetic test (addition task) for one hour without break. The stimulation consisted primarily of the subject's own uninterrupted activity. In both conditions recordings of performance level and psychophysiological changes were made before and after the task. With regard to the psychophysiological changes evoked by both conditions, measures of RT (to visual and auditory stimuli) and electrodermal activity (EDA) were under control. Let us concentrate on the latter measure. Changes in EDA, expressed in skin resistance units, were recorded continuously (at 1-minute intervals) throughout the experiment. For diagnosing reactivity the method known as the slope of RT curve (see Nebylitsyn, 1972; Strelau, 1983a) was used. Altogether 163 high-school students (males aged 17 to 19 years) were investigated. From this group 18 high and 17 low reactives were isolated.

The results obtained by Klonowicz suggest that under the poor-stimulation conditions, high-reactive subjects perform better than low-reactive ones, as chiefly reflected in the smaller number of errors (i.e., missing the signals). Under more stimulating demands (addition task), both groups showed the same level of performance.

Very distinct differences were recorded in the subjects' psychophysiological functioning under the two experimental conditions with regard to EDA. When the vigilance task was performed (poor stimulation), high-reactive subjects were relaxed, as indicated by their increased skin resistance; low-reactive subjects exhibited symptoms of increased activation, as reflected in their reduced skin resistance (see Figure 8.4A). As the experiment progressed, the differences between high and low reactives gradually increased, finally to reach the level of statistically significance ($t = 2.64$; $p < .05$).

As shown in Figure 8.4B the situation is exactly reversed under highly stimulating conditions. The curve representing the EDA of high-reactive subjects indicates their increased activation, while the graph of the low-reactive ones fails to reveal any psychophysiological changes under this condition. Here again the differences between both groups are very distinct and increasing with the progress of the experiment ($t = 2.89$; $p < 0.05$).

In conclusion, it may be stated that the data obtained by Klonowicz support our expectations that the psychophysiological costs under highly stimulating conditions are more pronounced in high reactives, whereas low-reactive subjects pay more costs in situations characterized by low stimulation.

As it is well known, long lasting psychophysiological changes developed under a chronic lack of equilibrium between the stimulative value of demands and the individual's capacity to cope with them lead to different psychosomatic diseases. In a study conducted by Jastrzębska, Nowakowska, and Strelau (1974) we were able to show that patients suffering from gastric or duodenum ulcers differed significantly from the control group (pair-matched healthy individuals) in such parameters as: reactivity, extraversion-introversion, type of energy release, and tolerance to stress in a problem-

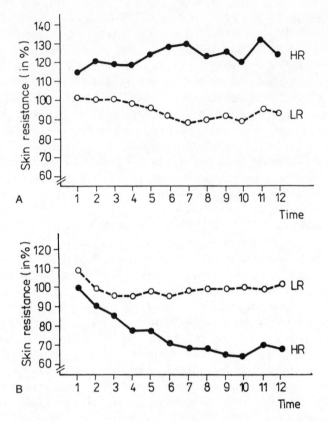

Figure 8.4. Skin resistance curves during vigilance (A) and addition (B) tasks as percent of the pre-work level (taken from Klonowicz, 1974).

solving situation. These differences were expressed in: (a) higher reactivity, (b) higher level of neuroticism, (c) lower tolerance to stress, (d) predominance of introvertive patterns, and (e) a tendency to react to tension by visceral activity.

The data were obtained from a total number of 100 subjects of both sexes (50 patients and 50 healthy individuals aged 20 to 50 years). Reactivity was measured by means of the STI, and extraversion-introversion with the Eysenck's MPI. Tolerance to stress, as well as the kind of tension release, were estimated on the basis of specially developed questionnaires.

Very recently a study conducted by Eliasz and Wrześniewski (in press) on over 1,000 high-school students shows evidence that the development of Type A behavior, to be met in both high- and low-reactive individuals, proceeds differently depending on the level of reactivity. In high-reactive students, Type A behavior pattern, being in essence very stimulating, develops under high psychophysiological costs. This is expressed, among other things, by a high level of anxiety. In low-reactive students, the Type A behavior pattern fits well with their high capacity for stimulation demands. Thus the psychophysiological costs of developing Type A, measured in this study by the level of anxiety, are lower for these individuals.

The examples presented seem to be unequivocal in supporting the hypothesis that reactivity is one of the temperament dimensions to be considered in determining the level of psychophysiological costs paid when the equilibrium of stressors and the individual's capability to cope with them is disturbed.

Coping with Stress and Individual Differences in Reactivity

The style and/or strategies of coping with stressors of too high or too low stimulative values have been subject to investigation in several experiments and field studies.

In regard to the strategies of behavior, it follows from the RTT that HR individuals should be inclined to develop relatively unstimulating strategies of behavior. In turn, low-reactive individuals will develop strategies of behavior that ensure stimulation of high intensity. High-reactive individuals will avoid situations that evoke strong emotional tension, that is, they avoid risk. This in turn provides for the development of a risk-avoidance strategy of action. The opposite occurs in individuals with a low level of reactivity. For these individuals the situation of risk is a desirable one because of its high stimulative value. This results in the development of a risky strategy of action. On the basis of these considerations we (Przymusiński & Strelau, 1986), adopted the following hypothesis in one of our experiments aimed at studying individual differences in decision making: individuals who prefer risk over probability in decision making in gambling situations (risk-takers) are characterized by temperamental traits that refer to a high demand of stimulation. In individuals who prefer probability over risk in the same situations (risk-avoiders), there is a dominance of temperamental traits that express a low need for stimulation.

Among 267 subjects (males and females aged from 17 to 21 years) 82 were selected as having consistent preferences in strategies to cope with risk—40 risk-takers and 42 risk-avoiders. The preferences were estimated on the basis of decision making in five gambling situations. In all of the games (which were of the same type), the subject had to choose one of the seven alternatives with probabilities of winning, ranging from one-in-eight to seven-in-eight. The skew coefficient (SC), which expresses the preference with respect to probabilities was used as the measure of the subject's preferences.

In order to measure temperament/personality traits, Eysenck's MPI, Spielberger's STAI, Thurstone's TTS, Strelau's STI, and Cattell's 16PF inventories have been administered.

The results show that among the 30 traits being investigated there are eight (see Table 8.1) that differentiate risk-takers and risk-avoiders. After factor analyzing them by means of the centroid method, we separated two factors as shown in Table 8.1. The highest loading in Factor I has reactivity

Table 8.1. Centroid Factor Matrix of Temperament Traits Which Differentiate Risk-Taking Decisions*

Traits	Factor Loadings	
	Factor I	Factor II
Strength of excitation (STI)	0.782	0.352
Mobility of NS (STI)	0.728	0.098
Vigorous (TTS)	0.631	−0.112
Impulsive (TTS)	0.702	0.187
Ego strength (16PF)	0.408	0.581
Dominance (16PF)	0.577	0.130
Paranoid suspicion (16PF)	−0.071	−0.482
Guilt proneness (16PF)	−0.465	−0.661

*From Przymusiński and Strelau, 1986.

Table 8.2. Proportion of Subjects in Relation to the Ratio of Auxiliary Actions (AA) to Basic Actions (BA) and Level of Reactivity*

Ratio of AA to BA	HR	LR	Total Number of Subjects
0–1.00	7	23	30
1.01–4.67	36	22	58
Total number of subjects	43	45	88

*From Strelau, 1983a.
$\chi^2 = 11.90$; $p < 0.01$.

and thereafter mobility of behavior as measured by STI, vigorousness (TSS), and impulsivity (TTS). These temperamental traits are strongly bound with the energetic characteristic of behavior.

The results of this study support the data obtained in one of the former experiments (Kozłowski, 1977) conducted in our laboratory, where it was shown that among risk-takers there are statistically significant more low-reactive and emotionally stable individuals as compared with risk-avoiders. Among the latter, high-reactive and neurotic individuals predominate.

Some of the richest empirical evidence collected in our laboratory refer to the relationships between reactivity and style of action. The reasons to search for these dependencies have been presented above. In almost all our studies, independent of the population and type of task under investigation, the results show that for high-reactive individuals the adjunctive style of action dominates (predominance of auxiliary activity over the basic one), whereas low-reactive individuals have a balanced ratio between both types of activities or the basic ones dominate over auxiliary activities (the straightforward style of action). The ratio of auxiliary actions (AA) to basic actions (BA) estimated in one of our experiments (see Strelau, 1983a) is presented in Table 8.2.

As can be seen, the low ratio of AA to BA (i.e., only a small number of auxiliary actions are or nothing performed) is typical for low-reactive subjects, whereas a high ratio of AA to BA, a dominance of AA over BA, is characteristic for high reactives. The results were obtained in the case when a so-called heuristic instruction was given in order to solve a construction task, the aim of which was to form an eyelet in a 2.5×2.5 cm square of self-adhesive plaster.

In the experiment two types of instruction were used in order to regulate the ratio of auxiliary and basic actions: the heuristic instruction, in which only the final goal was described and the subject was allowed to organize the activity in his/her own way by using optional methods of work; the algorithmic instruction, which consisted of describing not only the goal of the task, but also the operations in the order they had to be performed. The algorithmic instruction forces the subject to perform many auxiliary actions whereas the heuristic instruction gives the subject greater freedom to organize the functional structure of activity in his/her own way.

After solving the construction task under both types of instruction, a situation was arranged that allowed the subjects to choose whether they preferred to work further with the algorithmic or heuristic instruction. The results were according to our expectations. High-reactive individuals preferred to work under the algorithmic instruction, whereas among low-reactive individuals the heuristic instruction was chosen more often. These differences were statistically significant (see Strelau, 1983a). When the subjects had to work under conditions that did not allow them to use the style of action co-determined by their level of reactivity, a significant decrease in performance was obtained (see Klonowicz, 1984; Strelau, 1983a).

Mündelein (1982) conducted an experiment to study, among other things, the interrelation between level of reactivity and style of action; the latter was studied in laboratory conditions similar to the natural setting of an insurance agent working within a computer system. The task of the subject, playing the role of the agent, was to calculate the amount of compensation for clients suffering loss. The subject used the computer system, where all information needed to make the final decision was stored. The experiment lasted 3 hours. The basic actions included collecting and processing information and decision making. The subjects were additionally informed that the computer system, also used by people working in other offices, might become overloaded and that this could be checked by pressing the button labeled "system." If thereby informed that the computer was overloaded, the subject, to avoid unexpected disturbances, could press the button marked "priority" to insure undisturbed computer operation for a given period. Pressing the buttons "system" and "priority" is a typical auxiliary action, as the aim of it consists of protecting the basic actions against possible disturbances.

In regard to reactivity, individuals were selected for this experiment on the basis of the STI and by means of the slope of RT among 72 subjects of both sexes and ranging in age from 18 to 55 years. Only those subjects who

Table 8.3. Number of Auxiliary Actions Performed by High- and Low-Reactive Individuals*

Number of Auxiliary Action	Subjects	
	LR	HR
Pressing button "system"	46.8	61.9 [†]
Pressing button "priority"	13.6	15.2
Pressing button "system"/min	0.27	0.37[†]
Pressing button "priority"/min	0.08	0.09[†]

* Adapted from Mündelein, 1982.
[†] $p < 0.05$.

received a consistent diagnosis of reactivity based on both methods were considered. As a result, 22 low-reactive and 24 high-reactive subjects were separated.

As can be seen from Table 8.3, a significant difference exists between high- and low-reactive individuals in the number of auxiliary actions performed in favor of HR subjects. This result is in concert with our own studies and supports the hypothesis that the style of action plays an important role in regulating the stimulative value of demands the individual is confronted with, and this role is different depending on the level of reactivity.

The theoretical arguments, as well as the empirical evidence, which refer mainly to the relationship between stress and reactivity presented in this chapter, should be regarded as one of the many ways in which stress may be studied from the perspective of the individual differences approach.

Acknowledgment. This work has been financed by the Minister of Science and Higher Education (Grant: RPBP. III. 25)

References

Appley, M.H., & Trumbull, R. (1967). On the concept of psychological stress. In M.H. Appley & R. Trumbull (Eds.), *Psychological stress: Issues in research.* New York: Appleton-Century-Crofts.

Brebner, J. (in press). Personality factors in stress and anxiety. In C.D. Spielberger, I.G. Sarason, & J. Strelau (Eds.), *Stress and anxiety*, Vol. 12. Washington, DC: Hemisphere Publishing Corporation.

Broverman, D.M., Klaiber, E.L., Vogel, W., & Kobayashi, Y. (1974). Short-term versus long-term effects of adrenal hormones on behavior. *Psychological Bulletin, 81*, 672–694.

Chan, K.B. (1977). Individual differences in reactions to stress and their personality and situational determinants: Some implications for community mental health. *Social Science and Medicine, 11*, 89–103.

Cox, T. (1978). *Stress.* London: Macmillan Press.

Danilova, N.N. (1985). *Functional states: Mechanisms and diagnosis.* Moscow: Moscow University Press (in Russian).

Eliasz, A. (1981). *Temperament a system regulacji stymulacji* [Temperament and the Stimulation-regulating System]. Warszawa: Państwowe Wydawnictwo Naukowe.

Eliasz, A. (1985). Mechanisms of temperament: Basic functions. In J. Strelau, F. Farley, & A. Gale (Eds.), *The biological bases of personality and behavior: Theories, measurement techniques, and development*, Vol. 1. Washington, DC: Hemisphere Publishing Corporation.

Eliasz, A., & Wrześniewski, K. (in press). *Ryzyko chorób psychosomatycznych: środowisko i temperament a "Wzór zachowania A"* [Psychosomatic disease risk: Environment, temperament and Type A behavior pattern]. Warszawa: Państwowe Wydawnictwo Naukowe.

Endler, N.S., & Magnusson, D. (Eds.). (1976). *Interactional psychology and personality*. Washington, DC: Hemisphere Publishing Corporation.

Eysenck, H.J. (1967). *The biological basis of personality*. Springfield, IL: Thomas.

Eysenck, H.J. (1970). *The structure of human personality*. London: Methuen.

Eysenck, H.J. (1981a). General features of the model. In H.J. Eysenck (Ed.), *A model for personality*. Berlin: Springer-Verlag.

Eysenck, H.J. (Ed.). (1981b). *A model for personality*. Berlin: Springer-Verlag.

Fenz, W.D. (1975). Strategies for coping with stress. In I.G. Sarason & C.D. Spielberger (Eds.), *Stress and anxiety*, Vol. 2. Washington, DC: Hemisphere Publishing Corporation.

Friedman, M., & Rosenman, R.H. (1974). *Type A behavior and your heart*. New York: Knopf.

Glass, D.C., & Singer, J.E. (1972). *Urban stress: Experiments on noise and social stressors*. New York: Academic Press.

Gray, J.A. (Ed.). (1964). *Pavlov's typology*. Oxford: Pergamon Press.

Hebb, D.O. (1955). Drives and the C.N.S. (conceptual nervous system). *Psychological Review, 62*, 243–254.

Jastrzębska, A., Nowakowska, J., & Strelau, J. (1974). Cechy temperamentalne, odporność na stres a etiopatogeneza choroby wrzodowej [Temperamental traits, resistance to stress, and etiopathogenesis of gastric ulcer]. In J. Strelau (Ed.), *Rola cech temperamentalnych w działaniu*. Wrocław: Ossolineum.

Klonowicz, T. (1974). Reactivity and fitness for the occupation of operator. *Polish Psychological Bulletin, 5*, 129–136.

Klonowicz, T. (1984). *Reaktywność a funkcjonowanie człowieka w różnych warunkach stymulacyjnych* [Reactivity and human functioning in various stimulation conditions]. Wrocław: Ossolineum.

Klonowicz, T. (1985). Temperament and performance. In J. Strelau (Ed.), *Temperamental bases of behavior: Warsaw studies on individual differences*. Lisse, The Netherlands: Swets & Zeitlinger.

Klonowicz, T. (1987). Reactivity and the control of arousal. In J. Strelau & H.J. Eysenck (Eds.), *Personality dimensions and arousal*. New York: Plenum Press.

Kobasa, S.C. (1979). Stressful life events, personality and health: An inquiry into hardiness. *Journal of Personality and Social Psychology, 37*, 1–11.

Kozłowski, C. (1977). Demand for stimulation and probability preferences in gambling decisions. *Polish Psychological Bulletin, 8*, 67–73.

Krohne, H.W., & Rogner, J. (1982). Repression-sensitization as a central construct in coping research. In H.W. Krohne & L. Laux (Eds.), *Achievement, stress, and anxiety*. New York: Hemisphere/McGraw-Hill.

Lacey, J.I. (1967). Somatic response patterning and stress: Some revisions of activation theory. In M.H. Appley & R. Trumbull (Eds.), *Psychological stress: Issues in research*. New York: Appleton-Century-Crofts.

Laux, L., & Vossell, G. (1982). Theoretical and methodological issues in achievement-related stress and anxiety research. In H.W. Krohne & L. Laux (Eds.), *Achievement, stress, and anxiety*. New York: Hemisphere/McGraw-Hill.

Lazarus, R.S. (1966). *Psychological stress and the coping process*. New York: McGraw-Hill.

Lazarus, R.S. (1967). Cognitive and personality factors underlying threat and coping. In M.H. Appley & R. Trumbull (Eds.), *Psychological stress: Issues in research*. New York: Appleton-Century-Crofts.

Lundberg, U. (1982). Psychophysiological aspects of performance and adjustment to stress. In H.W. Krohne & L. Laux (Eds.), *Achievement, stress, and anxiety*. New York: Hemisphere/McGraw-Hill.

Lundberg, U., & Frankenhaeuser, M. (1978). Psychophysiological reactions to noise as modified by personal control over stimulus intensity. *Biological Psychology, 6*, 51– 59.

Magnusson, D. (1982). Situational determinants of stress: An interactional perspective. In L. Goldberger & S. Bresnitz (Eds.), *Handbook of stress*. New York: Free Press.

Matysiak, J. (1980). *Różnice indywidualne w zachowaniu zwierząt w świetle koncepcji zapotrzebowania na stymulację* [Individual differences in animal behavior in light of the theory of stimulation requirement]. Wrocław: Ossolineum.

McGrath, J.E. (1970a). A conceptual formulation for research on stress. In J.E. McGrath (Ed.), *Social and psychological factors in stress*. New York: Holt, Rinehart & Winston.

McGrath, J.E. (1970b). Major methodological issues. In J.E. McGrath (Ed.), *Social and psychological factors in stress*. New York: Holt, Rinehart & Winston.

McGrath, J.E. (1970c). Settings, measures, and themes: An integrative review of some research on social-psychological factors in stress. In J.E. McGrath (Ed.), *Social and psychological factors in stress*. New York: Holt, Rinehart & Winston.

McGrath, J.E. (1982). Methodological problems in research on stress. In H.W. Krohne & L. Laux (Eds.), *Achievement, stress, and anxiety*. New York: Hemisphere/ McGraw-Hill.

Meichenbaum, D. (1977). *Cognitive-behavior modification: An integrative approach*. New York: Plenum Press.

Mischel, W. (1969). Continuity and change in personality. *American Psychologist, 24*, 1012–1018.

Monat, A., & Lazarus, R.S. (1985). *Stress and coping: An anthology* (2nd ed.). New York: Columbia University Press.

Morris, L.W. (1979). *Extraversion and introversion: An interactional perspective*. Washington, DC: Hemisphere Publishing Corproation.

Mündelein, H. (1982). *Simulierte Arbeitssituation an Bildschirmterminals: Ein Beitrag zu einer ökologisch orientierten Psychologie*. Frankfurt/Main: Fischer Verlag.

Nebylitsyn, V.D. (1972). *Fundamental properties of the human nervous system*. New York: Plenum Press.

Opton, E.M., & Lazarus, R.S. (1967). Personality determinants of psychophysiological response to stress: A theoretical analysis and an experiment. *Journal of Personality and Social Psychology, 6*, 291–303.

Pavlov, I.P. (1951–1952). *Complete works* (2nd ed.). Moscow & Leningrad: SSSR Academy of Sciences (in Russian).

Przymusiński, R., & Strelau, J. (1986). Temperamental traits and strategies of decision-making in gambling. In A. Angleitner, A. Furnham, & G. van Heck (Eds.), *Personality psychology in Europe: Current trends and controversies*, Vol. 2. Lisse, The Netherlands: Swets & Zeitlinger.

Schalling, D. (1976). Anxiety, pain, and coping. In I.G. Sarason & C.D. Spielberger (Eds.), *Stress and anxiety*, Vol. 3. Washington, DC: Hemisphere Publishing Corporation.

Schönpflug, W. (1982). Aspiration level and causal attribution. In H.W. Krohne & L. Laux (Eds.), *Achievement, stress, and anxiety*. New York: Hemisphere/McGraw-Hill.

Schulz, P., & Schönpflug, W. (1982). Regulatory activity during states of stress. In H.W. Krohne & L. Laux (Eds.), *Achievement, stress, and anxiety*. New York: Hemisphere/McGraw-Hill.

Selye, H. (1956). *The stress of life*. New York: McGraw-Hill.

Selye, H. (1975). *Stress without distress*. New York: New American Library.

Selye, H. (1982). History and present status of the stress concept. In L. Goldberger & S. Breznitz (Eds.), *Handbook of stress: Theoretical and clinical aspects*. New York: Free Press.

Strelau, J. (1982). Biologically determined dimensions of personality or temperament? *Personality and Individual Differences*, *3*, 355–360.

Strelau, J. (1983a). *Temperament—personality—activity*. London: Academic Press.

Strelau, J. (1983b). A regulative theory of temperament. *Australian Journal of Psychology*, *35*, 305–317.

Strelau, J. (1985). Diversity of personality dimensions based on arousal theories: Need for integration. In J.T. Spence & C.E. Izard (Eds.), *Motivation, emotion, and personality*. Amsterdam: North Holland.

Strelau, J. (Ed.). (1986). *Temperamental bases of behavior: Warsaw studies on individual differences*. Lisse, The Netherlands: Swets & Zeitlinger.

Strelau, J. (1987a) The concept of temperament in research on personality. *European Journal of Personality*, *1*, 107–117.

Strelau, J. (1987b). Personality dimensions based on arousal theories: Search for integration. In J. Strelau & H.J. Eysenck (Eds.), *Personality dimensions and arousal*. New York: Plenum Press.

Strelau, J. (in press). Individual differences in tolerance to stress: The role of reactivity. In C.D. Spielberger, I.G. Sarason, & J. Strelau (Eds.), *Stress and anxiety*, Vol. 12. Washington, DC: Hemisphere Publishing Corporation.

Strelau, J., & Eysenck, H.J. (Eds.). (1987). *Personality dimensions and arousal*. New York: Plenum Press.

Tomaszewski, T. (1978). *Tätigkeit und Bewusstsein: Beiträge zur Einführung in die polnische Tätigkeitpsychologie*. Weinheim & Basel, Switzerland: Beltz Verlag.

Weick, K.E. (1970). The "ess" in stress: Some conceptual and methodolgical problems. In J.E. McGrath (Ed.), *Social and psychological factors in stress*. New York: Holt, Rinehart & Winston.

Wundt, W. (1874). *Grundzüge der Physiologischen Psychologie*. Leipzig: Verlag von W. Engelmann.

Żmudzki, A. (1986). *Poziom reaktywności a powodzenie w trakcie startu u zawodników w podnoszeniu ciężarów* [Level of reactivity and success during competition in weight lifters]. Warszawa: Wydawnictwa Instytutu Sportu.

Author Index

Subject Index